The Handbook of Practice Developme

Also available:
Case Studies on Practice Development edited by James Dooher, Andrew Clark and John Fowler

The Handbook of
Practice Development

edited by
Andrew Clark, James Dooher and John Fowler

Quay
Books

Mark Allen
Publishing Ltd

Quay Books Division, Mark Allen Publishing Ltd
Jesses Farm, Snow Hill, Dinton, Nr Salisbury, Wiltshire, SP3 5HN

British Library Cataloguing-in-Publication Data
A catalogue record is available for this book

© Mark Allen Publishing Ltd 2001

ISBN 1 85642 168 6

Printed in the UK by The Cromwell Press, Trowbridge, Wiltshire

Contents

Section 3: The validation and replication of practice development

Acknowledgements

Our grateful thanks go to all contributors who despite busy lives managed to find space and time to contribute to this book. Special thanks must go to Rosemary Simpson who acted as critical reader.

About the editors and contributors

The editors have a wide experience in clinical, organisational and educational aspects of practice development and have invited a range of contributors to assist in the task of providing the first comprehensive guide to practice development.

Editors

Andrew Clark RMN, RGN, CPN Cert, FETC, ENB 955, DMS, MBA

Andrew has held a number of posts including community psychiatric nurse, clinical nurse manager and patient services manager and up until January 1999 was a practice development nurse in the East Midlands. He currently works independently as a part-time Lecturer at De Montfort University, as an external trainer and a clinical nurse within a number of organisations in the public and private sector. He was one of the main contributors to *The Handbook of Clinical Supervision — your questions answered.*

James Dooher RMN, FHE Cert Ed, Dip HCR, MA

James has worked in a variety of psychiatric settings and spent three years as a practice development nurse specialising in rehabilitation nursing before moving full-time to education. He has an interest in research, and practice development and is currently registered for a PhD. He is a full-time Senior Lecturer at De Montfort University School of Nursing and Midwifery. He was one of the main contributors to *The Handbook of Clinical Supervision — your questions answered.*

John Fowler RGN, RMN, RCNT, RNT, Dip N, Cert Ed, BA, MA

John has a varied background in nursing and nurse education. He is currently Programme Leader for the BSc (Hons) Health Care Practice Programme at De Montfort University. This encompasses a variety of post registration ENB Awards and the UKCC Specialist

Practitioner Qualification. He has a particular interest in clinical supervision and the development of practice. He was the editor of *The Handbook of Clinical Supervision — your questions answered.*

Contributors

The contributors are drawn from a wide range of specialities and backgrounds and their writing style, content and level are naturally different. While certain features of the text have been changed by the editors to provide continuity, we have tried hard to keep the style of the original contributor. Some of the chapters are therefore academic in style while others are free-flowing, adding diversity to the text.

Lee Beresford RMN, M MedSc

Lee has held several posts including that of practice development nurse and works for Mental Services in Huddersfield. He is currently seconded to the NHS Executive Northern and Yorkshire region. His professional interests include mental health care for the elderly, dementia care and staff education and training.

Richard Byrt RMN, RNMH, RGN, PhD, BSc (Hons)

Richard holds a joint post with Arnold Lodge Medium Secure Unit and De Montfort University in Leicester. He has experience within the health services as a service user, informal carer, volunteer and research student, and has worked as a nurse in a variety of settings, including three therapeutic communities. His specific interests include service between user participation and empowerment in health care and the links between nursing practice development and research.

Dawn Freshwater RN, BA (Hons), RNT, Dip Transpersonal Psychotherapy, PhD

Dawn had a diverse clinical background before moving into nurse education. She developed a lecturer practitioner post aimed at facilitating research and practice development. Her PhD study explored the use of reflection within nursing practice and she continues to have a particular interest in this subject. She is currently Course Leader to a Masters in Nursing course at Nottingham University.

Nigel Goodrich RGN, RMN, BSc (Hons)

Nigel trained as a psychiatric and general nurse and worked in orthopaedics for a number of years. He was responsible for the facilitation of research, evidence-based practice and professional development on a large orthopaedic unit. He then joined De Montfort University as a Senior Lecturer working with qualified staff undergoing post registration specialist qualifications. He is currently completing a Masters in Business Administration.

Silvia Ham-Ying RGN, RM, Dip N STD, RNT, BSc (Hons), MSc

Silvia had a varied clinical background before entering nurse education. She has considerable experience as a teacher and educational manager. She is currently responsible for the Continuing Professional Studies division of the School of Nursing and Midwifery at De Montfort University.

Mark Johnson BA (Hons), MA, PhD

Mark is a social scientist by background specialising in health care issues. He has a particular interest in the equality of health provision and is a Reader in Primary Care and Associate Director of the Mary Seacole Research Centre at De Montfort University.

Keith Todd RGN, ENB 199, Cert Ed, RNT

Keith worked for a number of years in a large accident and emergency department and was subsequently appointed as a Tutor to the A & E post basic course. He is currently Senior Lecturer with the Continuing Professional Studies division at De Montfort University and has particular interest in ethical and legal issues concerned with health care.

Denis Walsh RGN, RM, BA (Hons), MA

Denis worked as a midwife for a number of years before taking up a post of research and development officer within a large midwifery department. He is currently a Senior Lecturer in the midwifery division at De Montfort University.

Ann Jackson RMN, BA (Hons), MA

Ann worked as a qualified nurse in mental health and then worked as a research and practice development nurse pursuing a long interest in nursing research and innovative practice. She now works as an external facilitator for project-based practice development across a range of settings at the RCN institute. Her special interest is in women's mental health and anti-oppressive research methodology and practice.

Cathy McGargow RGN, RM, HV, MBA

Cathy is Executive Director and Chief Nursing Advisor for Leicestershire Health Authority. She has lead responsibility for partnership working, primary care group/trust development and performance management, aspects of health strategy and nursing issues. She is also an Honorary Senior Lecturer at Leicester University. She shares responsibility with the Director of Public Health for quality and clinical governance. She is a nurse, midwife and health visitor and has an interest in comparative health care and change management.

Dr Paul Pleasance RGN, ITU Cert, PGCE, RNT, M Ed, Ed D

Paul's clinical background is in intensive care and coronary care nursing. He has been involved in nursing education for 20 years and is currently External Liaison Co-Ordinator at the School of Nursing and Midwifery, De Montfort University. His doctorate explored the approaches to studying and learning adopted by students under-taking a Dip HE in Nursing and his major research interests remain in the field of nursing education.

Gail Scothern BSc (Hons) Combined Studies, MSc Clinical Psychology

Gail is a consultant clinical psychologist and has worked for a number of years within an elderly psychiatric service. Her interests include service evaluation and development, working with long term personality issues and discursive psychology.

Porsotam Leal MSc (Health Sciences), B Pharm (Hons), PGCE, PG Cert, PP, FAETC, MR Pharm

Porsotam is a clinical pharmacist and has worked in a number of settings. His interests include pharmacy process, patient care process and compliance and models of pharmacy management.

Paul Rigby RMN, BA (Hons), MA, Dip N, Dip Ad Ed

Paul has held a number of posts in psychiatry including lecturer practitioner and is currently a Senior Lecturer at De Montfort University. His professional interests centre around enduring mental health issues and the development of advanced practitioners.

Introduction

The Handbook of Practice Development provides a broad and comprehensive text for the busy practitioner. Written by a wide range of academics, clinical practitioners and strategic managers it provides a considerable insight into practice development. Dealing with issues such as accountability, education, clinical governance and supervision the handbook offers a valuable guide to all those involved in development of practice. Its companion, *Case Studies on Practice Development,* contains 23 reflective case studies of practice development written by practising clinicians. Together these books serve as a rich source of ideas, theories and real life experiences. The authors of each chapter have been chosen because of their particular knowledge, experience and expertise in their subject. The editors are grateful to all the contributors for being prepared to share their knowledge and experience in this way. The book is divided into three sections:

1. The concept of practice development.
2. The reality of implementing developments in practice.
3. The validation and replication of practice development.

An advantage of the book is that it does not need to be read in sequence starting with chapter one, each chapter, although relating to others within its section and the book as a whole, can be read in its own right. If you have a particular interest in accountability or clinical supervision go to those chapters first. As editors we hope you enjoy the book and find it a useful resource for your own practice and its development. Practice development, rather like swimming, will not occur by reading books about it and standing at the pool side looking on. However, jumping in at the deep end without first learning the basic swimming strokes can lead to disaster. This book, together with *Case Studies on Practice Development,* will inspire you to 'have a go' while at the same time giving you enough knowledge to know your limits and develop safely.

Conventions used throughout the book

For ease of reading a small number of conventions are used. 'Area' means ward, community team, trust, organisation, nursing home, department etc.

Where the convention 'she' is used as an alternative to constant repetition of practice development nurse, no slight on our male colleagues is intended!

Where the abbreviation PD appears it denotes practice development, PDN denotes practice development nurse.

Section 1:
The concept of practice development

1

The development of practice development

James Dooher

The mere acquisition of the necessary knowledge is easy. You will imbibe knowledge of your duties partly from direct teaching and from your handbook, but mainly you will soak it in from the daily experience of your lives. But over and above knowledge, far beyond it and more important, is character. It is character that counts, not cleverness, not even knowledge; capability and sympathy first and before all; grit and determination; integrity, loyalty, and uprightness; these are treasures that neither moth nor rust doth corrupt, and that thieves cannot break through and steal; those who have little can cultivate it into much, and those who have much can cultivate it into more. The life's work that you have chosen is arduous and trying beyond the work of most, but it has great compensations.

Campbell-Clark *et al*, 1923

If 'character' were the only attribute needed for a successful and dynamic health care career, survival would be assured for the majority of longsuffering professional providers in the UK. Qualifications, publications, manual dexterity, vision, technical skill, communication ability, interpersonal skill, personal integrity, social conformity and humour are all prerequisites to occupational success. Without a healthy combination of these attributes workers are vulnerable to the charges of incompetence and stagnation.

The concept of practice development means many things to many people. To some practitioners it is a threat that removes the comfort of the predictable week; to the manager it may be a stick to beat the workforce with; to the auditor it is an opportunity to measure workforce performance; to the patient it is another inconsistency in the care they receive; but to the visionary practitioner it is a means of liberating habitual routines, optimising resources and developing new strategies for care.

Liberation from the shackles of antiquated working procedure and policy may not be necessarily straightforward, and the abdication of one's responsibilities to provide innovative care may be seen as a passive and relatively comfortable option. The development of one's practice on the other hand, may be considered from two opposing perspectives. Firstly we may assume that as paid health care professionals we want to give a good service, and consequently strive to provide the best we can within our power. If a professional trying to provide the best (and generating radical ideas to develop practice) feels more open to criticism, then the likelihood of that person voicing their ideas reduces.

To be criticised for being no good at our job or too radical in our approach, is an issue we would all like to avoid, and the consequence results in cognitive dissonance. Cognitive dissonance can be explained as psychological discomfort or tension (Gross, 1988). The basis of this idea is that whenever an individual simultaneously holds two cognitions (thoughts) which are psychologically inconsistent, they experience dissonance.

Cognitions are *'the things a person knows about himself, about his behaviour and about his surroundings'* (Festinger, 1957) and any two cognitions can be:

Consonant or compatible (A implies B) A = Having a good idea that could improve practice B = I will be rewarded for voicing my good idea
Dissonant or incompatible (A implies not B, the obverse of A) A = Having a good idea that could improve practice B = I will be criticised for voicing my good idea and my career will be in jeopardy OR Irrelevant to each other

When an individual experiences this discomfort they are motivated to reduce it by achieving consonance, and change their attitude to reduce the dissonance. In this example health care professionals may either keep quiet or modify their thoughts and ideas to conform with the standard practice. The example also demonstrates that the anxiety created through the fear of criticism inhibits the creative process and consequently deprives the organisation or profession of the opportunity to consider development.

An example of when dissonance is likely to arise is if we have ideas about changing practice and also believe that we will be criticised for voicing those ideas. Assuming that we would rather not be criticised, the cognition, 'I have radical ideas that will improve care' is psychologically inconsistent with the cognition, 'voicing radical ideas is career suicide'. In this case the most effective (and perhaps the healthiest) way to reduce dissonance is to stop having ideas about improving practice. However most of us will seek out consistency in our cognition and, for example, we might:

* belittle the evidence about the career limiting aspects of challenging current practice
* associate with other radical thinkers and doers (eg. 'If so-and-so gets away with it, then it can't be very dangerous')
* have the idea but get a colleague to voice it (eg. load the gun but get someone else to fire it)
* make a virtue out of it by developing a romantic, daredevil image and flaunting danger by voicing ideas and challenging the status quo.

All these possible ways of reducing dissonance demonstrate that dissonance theory regards the human being not as a rational creature but as a rationalising one, attempting to appear rational both to others and to oneself. However, seeking out cognitive consistency may perhaps be counterproductive in terms of developing practice.

Secondly, practice development may be seen as a veiled managerial tool which organisations use covertly to embarrass their workforce, in order to provide an improved service at no additional cost, although alternatively the maintenance of the status quo may be legitimate for operational reasons. There have been some initiatives that have recognised the need for personal and professional development, and for nurses this would include the introduction of Post Registration Education and Practice (PREP) which ensures that nurses, midwives and health visitors receive a mandatory five days (or 35 hours) training every three years. This is supported by a continuing professional development standard (UKCC, 1999a) in which registered nurses are required to undertake a demonstrable process of continuing professional development. To meet this standard, the evidence to support professional growth and learning is collected in a personal professional profile. Compliance with these standards is mandatory for the maintenance of registration, and from April 2001 the UKCC will audit that compliance. This represents both carrot and stick, in the sense that the national body are actively encouraging professional growth, but if you cannot demonstrate that growth, they (United Kingdom Central Council) will not issue the licence to practise, and in effect interrupt or terminate a career in health.

The development of professional growth on an individual level is a prerequisite to the development of practice at a local level, however the transition between these two points is one that is differentiated by risk. There is very little professional risk associated with individual professional growth, although the development of practice is awash with personal, ethical, moral and professional liability. Employing organisations may have a vested interest in the smothering of innovation if it reduces the risk of litigation, however evidence-based interventions by default must emerge from a range of alternatives, and it is those alternatives which must be eliminated before the most successful option emerges.

The freedom to fail is one freedom that has not traditionally been seen as appropriate in professional health care, yet should be an integral part of innovation (Peters, 1993). If practice development is to be more than a regurgitation of bygone ideas, policies or procedures, the innovators themselves must be given permission to fail and try again. If this understanding is not reached then creativity will be stifled and clinical growth will undoubtedly be inhibited.

Failure is eschewed for a host of reasons including the explicit and implicit organisational fear of litigation, professional pride and the fear of finite resources being withdrawn from projects that do not get it right first time.

These factors have promulgated the craving for research and the understanding that if a practice is not evidence-based then it should not be considered. To work on one's gut feeling is not sufficient to risk resources, yet the very basis of research follows the development of a hypothesis which is essentially the researchers gut feeling, and the emergence of a question based on intuition. Verma and Beard (1981) described the hypothesis as a tentative proposition which is subject to verification and that in many cases the hypothesis is a hunch that the researcher has about the existence of a relationship between variables.

Changes in routine are often stressful, and the innovative practitioner will often face resistance in the form of dogmatic obstruction from colleagues. This obstruction may be overt, as in open up front objections, or covert resistance to change through a stated willingness to participate, but no real action to accompany the support. This reaction is often the result of absolutist thinking. Defined by Ostell and Oakland (1999), as a style of thinking which is believed to promote emotional distress, particularly anger, when people are confronted by situations which do not conform to their demands concerning what ought to happen. These are the result of an emotional investment and an attachment to practice or procedure which is precious to them. The obstructive colleague may have reached a plateau of understanding in relation to their duties, and should not necessarily be castigated for maintaining their views. The innovator must attempt to capitalise on what has already been achieved, celebrating the successes of the past, while attempting to engage obstructors with the notion of refining the original idea.

New and creative ideas are often dismissed by experienced colleagues before they have been given a fair hearing.

The development of practice as a phenomenon should recognise the importance of the innovation itself, as well as the need to persuade peers, managers and recipients of care that the change is worthwhile.

There are said to be four basic variables, that make a communication persuasive (Hovland *et al* 1953). These include:

♦ attractiveness
♦ credibility
♦ power
♦ similarity.

If the boundaries of clinical practice are to be pushed forward, then practice developers should consider these four factors in relation to both the desired outcome, and the perception others have of them as a person and a professional. These four factors are considered to be most persuasive when they come from individuals or groups who are attractive, credible, powerful or similar to the recipient of the communication.

In many cases innovation is driven from the professionals working at the bedside, and the ideas person may not have traditional forms of power such as hierarchical or financial responsibility. Commonly known as a 'bottom up' approach. Practice developers often rely on the power of clinical expertise rather than their hierarchical position in the organisation. The individual's plausibility in the clinical field, and the ability to convince through an evidence base is often the most powerful tool available. The attractiveness and personal charisma of the practice developer will also have an impact on the probability of success. This does not mean to say that practice developers need to be beauty contestants but rather that good ideas need to be delivered or presented with enthusiasm, optimism and a genuine desire to improve the situation. To develop the most persuasive case for change the presenter must highlight the added value their idea may bring. If this idea is within the scope of the organisation's mission statement or philosophy, then managers will immediately identify a similarity in terms of the goals and therefore be more likely to accept it.

Despite Hovland's ideas being almost fifty years old it is clear that these assertions are as relevant today as they were when first proposed, and that new innovations can capitalise on old ideas. In the Health Service Circular (HSC) *Better Health and Better Health Care,* the NHS Executive (1998a) made clear its intention to ensure that the recommended proposals would be implemented through partnership, and with an agreement to identify those best placed to lead on particular issues. Two months later in another HSC (NHS Executive, 1998b), it was recognised that the contribution of nurses, health visitors and midwives was 'vital and wide ranging', and acknowledged that these professions should provide the fulcrum on which the success of government policy would hinge. This should have provided a platform from which practice development nurses could bang their respective clinical drums. However, it seems that these agendas have been hijacked by others somewhere within the dissemination of power cascade.

The taking of risks is an issue that often contradicts professional stability.

Without doubt many interested health care professionals have inspirational ideas, that have the capacity to develop their particular area of practice, but are obstructed by the complexities of receiving organisational sanction to proceed. This notion does not propose that all wacky ideas should be translated into practice, but that creative thought should be both encouraged and considered.

Ratification to proceed following consideration should be on the basis of good faith and an organisational understanding that failure and learning are synonymous. Speculative attempts to improve a service or procedure must be framed in the context of ensuring safety for all concerned. Where safety is not at risk, ideas, however abstract or intangible, should be examined.

The gap between theory and practice, considered to be omnipresent, is a divide about which much has been written. The criticism for its existence is often levelled at the providers of education. The development of practice must be in tandem with the development of theory, with equal responsibility acknowledged by both sides.

2

What does a practice development nurse do?

Wendy Biddington

The essence of this job is described within the title. One element is the development of nurses' clinical skills while the other is to expand professional boundaries. Through role modelling it also involves maintaining one's own credibility as an up-to-date practitioner. My work in a variety of places such as the public, private and voluntary sectors and in different settings namely hospital, community and a nursing home has given me a wealth of experiences to draw upon. These experiences have proved invaluable and along with academic studies help me to bring a questioning and creative approach to practice development.

For the purpose of this chapter I asked colleagues what characteristics and skills they thought were needed to become a practice development nurse. Using their descriptions I will share my perceptions of the role.

Jack of all trades and possibly master of none?

A practice development nurse has to be something to everyone but not necessarily an expert in any one specialty. This might sound contentious to some but realistically it is impossible to be an expert in all the departments and areas of nursing in the two community hospitals in which I work. Through clinical governance there is a commitment to,

> *... improving the quality of services and safeguarding high standards of care by creating an environment in which excellence in clinical care will flourish.*

Department of Health, 1997

To become effective in the role, the practice development nurse needs to be the catalyst in this process. It may occur through having the skills to question what is observed, or through providing audit evidence or supporting staff as they plan and implement new initiatives. This requires confidence and assertiveness to speak out when skills or practice need changing. It is also important to acknowledge when one is unsure and being able to say, 'I don't know'. Building this sort of open relationship is about working in partnership.

Working in partnership

I wholeheartedly agree with the colleague who felt that working in partnership was a key characteristic to becoming a practice development nurse. Working in partnership involves not only nurses but the multi-disciplinary team, the patient, the carers and other agencies. It includes helping staff to find out about services or facilities or offering a more global view to a situation. Working in partnership also means responding to urgent situations and having a flexible personality to be able to put aside planned tasks for the new situation. The purpose of such partnerships is to achieve the best outcome for the patient. This approach encourages clinical effectiveness, ie. 'doing the right thing in the right way and at the right time for the right patient' (Royal College of Nursing, 1996).

An open office door where staff feel welcomed and able to discuss issues fosters partnerships. It also provides an opportunity for staff to reflect upon a particular event, reflection being a requirement in one's professional portfolio (UKCC, 1995a). Being tuned into this reflective and reviewing process is one way of promoting a learning culture.

A reviewer

This seemed a really good description of the sort of personality required for the role. One colleague described this as being a roving journalist. A journalist reports both good and bad news, investigates with tenacity and focus, questions, analyses, writes articles using modern technology, and all this within a code of conduct. The same sort of attributes are required of the practice development nurse with a code of conduct laid down by the UKCC (1992a). Sharing the good news can be demonstrated when affirming good practice, encouraging and using staff who have acquired new skills and being able to share in some of their successes. However, the role also requires sharing the bad news. This means that one is not always popular with staff especially if investigation shows a shortfall.

Because the role is multi-conceptual and multifaceted, tenacity and focus are required to deal with the job in hand. Invariably, a questioning approach results in one question leading to another. The ability to set objectives and time scales is a great asset and it avoids being overwhelmed by the demands of the job. Alongside this, the assertiveness to say 'no' is also a useful attribute. Investigative and analytical skills are also a key requirement. Being able to read policies or reports with an eye to detail and write concise and relevant responses are also essential skills of the practice development nurse. On a personal note, it was as a result of academic studies that I first really understood the importance of these skills.

Like a journalist the job requires getting out and about and meeting people. The news will not be unearthed by sitting in the office. One needs to listen to and talk to staff, to work alongside them and meet them where they are. This requires sensitivity to the clinical situation and knowledge of the real world of time restraints and staffing difficulties. The whole point of the reviewer analogy is the process of searching out information and communicating it.

A communicator

The skills needed here are not just giving information through the verbal or the written word, but to be interactive. Recognising how others are feeling, picking up cues about ideas, ensuring staff feel 'safe' to express opinions and listening attentively to staff are important. As a communicator, colleagues also included the need to convey to staff the feeling of being valued, and generate an encouraging and supportive culture where both praise and criticism are accepted. Much of the success in creating this culture will depend on diplomacy and negotiation.

Of course communication is a two-way process. I suspect that we can all relate the occasion when on the one hand we stand accused of not communicating and, on the other hand, staff expressing surprise that they need to reciprocate. Whatever the means, cultivating an effective communication system will help build relationships and trust. One also needs the ability to recognise where communications get blocked in the system to avoid the 'black holes' where information is 'lost'. Good communication skills are vital to the successful implementation of change.

The change agent

One nurse described the practice development nurse as being an innovator or someone who can make things happen. Being creative in developing clinical practice will inevitably result in change and change management. Change can be perceived as threatening and challenging with perhaps an implication that there is something wrong with present practice. To become effective as a change agent needs great patience, enthusiasm and energy. Encouraging and motivating staff is exciting but exhausting. For this reason developing good personal support networks and access to clinical supervision can help put things into perspective. Personally, I see this as part of the survival plan.

One colleague felt that tenacity was needed to become a practice development nurse, like a dog at a bone. While an interesting description, the dog will find it disappointing if the bone has no meat on it. A discerning attitude will help identify what is necessary and the key people who will help in the change process. Discernment will also help the individual to acknowledge if proposed changes are the result of a personal agenda or for the benefit of the community.

As a change agent one needs to take on a facilitative and enabling role. It is necessary to foster a culture in which it is implicit that all have a part to play in developing new ideas, in responding to and internalising change. The practice development nurse needs to be affirmative, democratic and nurturing in this process and act as a guide and resource for consultation, discussion and, in some instances, overseeing the process.

Being a resource

This requires a wide knowledge base which will have been acquired partly through life's experiences and partly through one's career, hence the description by an auxiliary who described this attribute as being a 'resource on legs'. Implicit in the role is the desire to search out information by tapping into the multitude of resources available. It is also about being aware of the political agenda as this has great influence on practice. Information gained then needs interpretation and to be shared with staff to help them understand the purpose and benefit of any development. This is part of the catalyst effect of the role already mentioned.

Staff who are given the opportunity to test the waters with a new project and have the appropriate resources can become the springboards for innovative practice.

Along with providing support, the practice development nurse needs the skills to know when to be actively involved and when to stand back and help others to take ownership and credit. Being a resource also means having the confidence to make phone calls to find out information and build networks. The phrase, 'I can't but I know a man who can' is about using those networks. As one's own areas of expertise become known this process can be reciprocated. Being involved in the change process and being a resource to staff is very time-consuming. Planning and setting objectives were also felt by colleagues to be key requirements for the job.

A planner

Much of the work of the hospital practice development nurse is self-generated and requires good organisation to meet objectives. It is necessary to use one's initiative, be comfortable working alone and to cope with sometimes feeling isolated. It is a senior post involving both management and nursing which occasionally results in conflicting opinions and ideas. As a planner one needs to see an issue in context with all the other issues and to set realistic time scales and goals for development and achievement. Failing to do so will result in all feeling demoralised.

There are many initiatives being developed at any one time and the practice development nurse needs to keep them all in mind. A colleague likened this to being a juggler with each ball or initiative having its own place and importance in the overall scheme of things. Being able to flip quickly and easily from one subject to another and have speedy recall is also helpful in this juggling act. Such mental flexibility is described by Pedler *et al* (1986) as a 'helicopter mind'. In addition, being astute to organisational influences and having a working knowledge of well tested management strategies such as team dynamics (Belbin, 1981), being a change agent (Lancaster and Lancaster, 1982), and time management (Pedler *et al,* 1986) will all help the planning process.

Complementing all these skills to promote clinical development are the skills and abilities needed to create a learning culture.

Creating a learning environment

In becoming a practice development nurse one needs an interest in teaching and the principle of life-long learning. Being creative in developing a successful learning environment is described by Biddington (1996) and encouraging staff to acknowledge that opportunistic and informal learning is as valid as formalised teaching, will help generate this culture.

An integral part of the learning environment is maintaining one's own clinical skills and being seen as both the teacher and the student, a novice in some things and an expert in others (Benner, 1984). This approach is perhaps an important way to *'integrate theory and practice in education settings and practice areas'* (NHS Executive, 1998c). It is certainly an approach which will help close the theory/practice gap especially if there are good links between hospital and university.

Working within a learning culture promotes professional development and progression of personal development plans. The practice development nurse needs to facilitate staff to achieve this and develop their competencies within the *Scope of Practice* (UKCC, 1992b) A healthy interest in one's own professional development is also important. This may include undertaking a research project or further studies or sharing good practice through writing journal articles. One colleague described this as maintaining 'street cred'.

Learning can also be encouraged through maintaining close links with departments, being interested in staff and taking their enquiries seriously. Therefore one needs an interest in people and a commitment to them.

Accountable

The practice development nurse is accountable for professional practice. One of the skills needed in this post is to help staff understand that accountability should be seen in terms of doing one's best for the patient as a professional. At present it appears staff perceive that accountability is for the benefit of the UKCC and to avoid their punitive actions.

Another aspect of accountability is to be able to evaluate the effectiveness of the role. Developing a system to substantiate how and why clinical practice has changed, how nurses have developed professionally and how as an individual one has developed is essential. This will help to provide demonstrable and measurable evidence that the investment in this role is worthwhile.

Conclusion

So what does it take to become a practice development nurse? Colleagues talked of many skills and attributes making the Jack of all trades description seem very appropriate. To become successful in developing clinical skills it would appear one needs an investigative personality which will uncover good and bad practice and be the catalyst for change and improvement. Good communications, collaborative working, good planning and making use of available resources will help achieve a successful outcome. Interpersonal skills play an important part in making staff feel valued, consulted and encouraged to have a go at new ideas.

In expanding professional development the practice development nurse needs to be available to staff as a resource from a sound knowledge base and through networking. Creating a learning environment will increase knowledge and competencies and help staff to achieve their potential.

I do not imagine that I have all these skills but do have an organised, questioning and inventive personality. I hope this is complemented by sound clinical skills, empathy with staff and a sense of humour, keeping me credible, nursing focused and human. The wider vision of expanded roles and professional development are skills acquired through gaining confidence, through knowledge of accountability and through the experiences of life-long learning.

In varying degrees all nurses have the attributes mentioned in this chapter. However, most require someone in the role of the practice development nurse to be the catalyst in progressing clinical and professional development.

3

How can I become a clinical expert?

Paul Rigby

Being identified as a clinical expert is perhaps something to which most nurses would not readily lay claim. However, the development of clinical expertise is crucial to the provision of effective patient care. The issue of whether the characteristics of experts are developed or inherited remains a contentious one (Ericsson and Smith, 1991). Nevertheless, it has been, and still is, popular within nursing to accept that experience contributes significantly towards the development of expertise (Benner, 1984). The use of intuition and experience are features which, it is still argued, distinguish 'experts' from their 'proficient' and 'competent' counterparts (Benner and Tanner, 1987). Other key features include a willingness to continually critically evaluate clinical practice and the ability to work and develop within a culture of dynamic change.

It is important to note that while experience is important in the development of expertise, it is not simply a matter of time serving in clinical practice, but also involves for the practitioner the continuous development of meaningful knowledge and skills.

It is not possible to develop clinical expertise without adopting a questioning approach and as practitioners we need to be continually examining our clinical practice and asking the following questions:

Is my nursing care effective?
Is my nursing practice supported by sound evidence?
How can I demonstrate that I am clinically effective?
Does evidence exist that will help me improve my practice and if so, where can I find it?

The pursuit of clinical effectiveness has now become a political as well as a professional goal, and providers of health care are now responsible for ensuring that their nursing practice is based upon firm evidence supporting its success (DoH, 1998a). Phrases such as clinical effectiveness have now become part of everyday language for nurses and describe,

... the extent to which specific clinical interventions when deployed in the field for a particular patient or population do what they are intended to do – that is maintain and improve

health and secure the greatest possible health gain from the available resources.

NHS Executive, 1996

Or to put it more simply, doing the right thing, in the right way, for the right patient at the right time (Garbett, 1998). The concept of evidence-based practice (EBP), has grown from the global desire for clinical effectiveness, in which clinicians use the best evidence available to guide their clinical decision-making. There are a variety of steps that are necessary prior to getting to the stage where best evidence is utilised in clinical practice and these involve the following:

+ developing a culture that questions clinical practice
+ critically examining your practice and identifying relevant issues/questions etc
+ searching for evidence that are of relevance to these issues/questions
+ analysing the evidence you find
+ applying the relevant findings to practice
+ evaluating the success of your implementation.

What does each of these stages involve for the practitioner?

Developing a culture that questions practice

The development of an open and honest environment in which clinical care issues are discussed critically is essential towards fostering clinical effectiveness. There exist many opportunities for practitioners to question clinical care issues; during handover/ reports, case conferences/presentations, when planning and evaluating plans of care or simply discussing ideas with colleagues. The clinical environment has to support and nourish a questioning approach for practitioners to be able to question practice with confidence. Practitioners themselves have to be willing to learn and accept that their clinical practice needs to continually develop if it is to remain dynamic. Often the impetus for changes in our own practice, certainly in the formative stages of our careers, comes initially from other practitioners whom we see as good role models. Working alongside skilled, experienced practitioners can be very beneficial in terms of developing the confidence to question what are often very established methods of care delivery.

Critically examining clinical practice

The critical examination of your clinical practice is vital to developing clinical effectiveness and reflective practice is an essential tool in this process. Reflective practice groups actively encourage the sharing of ideas, concerns, questions, challenges and celebrations of practice and can be an effective way of supporting practitioners' reflections (Andrews, 1996). Developing skills of reflection and having the confidence to examine and, ideally, share these examples with others can be very beneficial towards maintaining a dynamic approach to nursing practice development.

Searching for evidence

What is the right sort of evidence and where can you find it? The quality of information that is accepted as 'best evidence' is a source of increasing debate, ie. is it only research studies using quantitative methods that are acceptable or are studies using qualitative methods equally as valid? There is clearly a hierarchy of accepted evidence which has randomised control trials (RCTs) at the top and a personal account of experience/case study at the bottom (Sullivan, 1998). While the rigour of the evidence is important, there are within many areas of nursing practice a distinct absence of RCTs relating to key issues. While it is important to identify the most relevant and rigorous evidence to support clinical practice, it is both necessary and desirable to be flexible in your approach to what constitutes 'evidence'. Who knows, you may choose to conduct your own research to add weight to the evidence that already exists.

There is a wealth of information available published and unpublished; including journal articles, books, research reports and the internet.

Analysing the evidence

Once you have found the right material, it is important to analyse it to identify what is relevant and worthwhile to your particular clinical practice issue. Certainly, a working knowledge of research methodology is highly desirable here. It will enable you to quickly identify not only the strength of the research-based work that you find, but also the potential for areas of future research that you may wish to explore or that you identify as being absent from the existing evidence. Discussing your findings with colleagues either informally or through a journal club is important here and issues such as the strength of the research design and the applicability of the published work to your own clinical field will need to be addressed.

Applying the evidence

The whole process of critically examining your practice is pointless if it does not lead on some occasions at least, to a change in nursing care. It may be that you discover evidence that supports your current practice; equally, you may well identify evidence that suggests changes to your practice. Such changes may be in relation to individual practice initially and then may lead to changes in a broader sense through the development of clinical standards or care pathways.

Sharing your findings and expertise with others is essential to maintaining a critical perspective towards clinical practice. This can be achieved in a variety of ways by student/peer supervision, formal and informal teaching opportunities, participation in working groups and by publicising/publishing your work.

Evaluating the success of your implementation

Some thought will have to be given to the process of evaluating the success of implementing change in your clinical practice. This could be achieved by designing an evaluation tool or measure or, indeed, by the process of clinical audit. A more individual approach could be through reflections upon clinical practice which may be shared through a reflective practice group. Whatever method is chosen, it is important that clinical practice is not only based upon sound evidence, but that it is proved to be making a real difference to the quality of care provided and achieving what it is supposed to, to the satisfaction of all.

The importance of continuing professional development (CPD) to generating effective practice cannot be underestimated as both formal and informal educational opportunities can help to broaden the perspective in which we see our own particular specialities.

Case study

Shabana is a forty-two-year-old RMN, who has been qualified for twenty years and is currently working in a challenging behaviour unit for people with long term mental health problems.

Recently, a reflective practice group has commenced at the unit and after attending a few meetings, Shabana decides to volunteer to present a piece of reflective practice to the group. Her reflection focuses upon a verbal interaction with a client who has schizophrenia and in particular relates to the difficulties that can be encountered attempting to help somebody who is experiencing auditory hallucinations.

Shabana shares her reflection with the group and it generates discussion among her colleagues who have experienced similar challenges in their nursing practice. From this, Shabana decides to find out more about nursing interventions with people who are experiencing auditory hallucinations.

A visit to the local nursing library results in a literature search using electronic databases and Shabana now has a variety of journal articles to read concerning auditory hallucinations and the phenomenon of 'voice hearing'. Further to this, she discovers that there is a wealth of material particularly concerning user's perspectives on voice hearing on the internet, and accessing this gives her a new perspective.

Following her reading, and armed with new found knowledge, Shabana is keen to discuss her findings with other team members including the team psychologist who has a range of voice hearing assessments that she is willing to discuss with her.

Shabana's first attempts to utilise these assessments with clients that she has nursed for many years gives her a fresh insight into their symptoms and the coping mechanisms that they find most beneficial. From the client's perspective they value the quality time with Shabana and appreciate that someone is willing to talk to them about this particular aspect of their illness.

Fuelled by this experience, Shabana shares her ideas with her unit manager who encourages her to form a small working group to explore the possibility of using these assessments across the unit and to examine the impact that they may have to the quality of care provided overall.

Resulting from a lack of in-depth knowledge and understanding concerning auditory hallucinations, this example demonstrates that, given the right impetus, a critical examination of current clinical practice can lead, potentially, to significant changes in nursing practice and to a better quality service for service users.

Shabana becomes the driving force of this group and is soon hoping to access a formal training package in relation to psychosocial interventions and schizophrenia to improve her skill base.

The example of Shabana is a fairly simple one. It demonstrates a small step in a long process of developing one's clinical practice. Shabana had a wealth of clinical experience and it is all too easy to sit back relying on that experience and become complacent to the development of one's own practice. Being prompted by a supportive peer group Shabana 'bravely' reflects on her practice, reviews the current evidence, discusses possibilities with colleagues and develops her practice. Development of practice and development of clinical expertise becomes a journey, always moving in a forwards direction.

4

What is the role of reflection in practice development?

Dr Dawn Freshwater

Introduction

Nursing, along with other professions, has seen an increasing interest in the potential of reflection as a learning tool and as a means of integrating the theory and practice of nursing (Freshwater, 1998; Rolfe, 1998; Osbourne, 1996; Atkins and Murphy, 1993). A simple example of this can be seen in the case study on Shabana in *Chapter 3*.

Referred to in the new strategy for Nursing, Midwifery and Health Visiting *Making a Difference* (DoH, 1999a), reflective practice values learning that takes place at work, that is learning through experience. Such learning includes insights gained from critical incidents, clinical supervision, peer review and audit processes. The potential of reflective practice for work-based learning is now well documented (Rolfe, 1998a; Johns, 1998; Johns and Freshwater, 1998) but what, more specifically, is the interface between reflection and practice development? It would appear that in the current climate there is a growing demand for nurses to maintain a closer compatibility between their espoused theories and their theories in action (Arygris and Schön, 1974) with increasing importance being placed on evidence-based practice and clinical effectiveness. This chapter explores the links between some of these contemporary issues and practice development. The aim is to explore, albeit briefly, some of the ways in which reflection and reflective practice may be actively engaged in as part of practice development and its influence on practice innovations, research and evidence-based practice. It is proposed that a commitment to developing practice necessitates a reflective and effective practitioner.

Reflective practice

The notion of reflective practice is a concept that is now much rehearsed in the nursing literature and as such will not be addressed in detail in this chapter. However, in attempting to understand the relationship between reflection, reflective practice and practice development it seems important to begin by defining some of the more popular interpretations of reflection. The basic purpose of reflection is to make sense of experience, definitions are flexible and dynamic, mirroring the process of learning from experience (Freshwater, 1998).

Johns (1995) for example interprets reflection as being,

... the practitioner's ability to access, make sense of and learn through work experience, to achieve more desirable, effective and satisfying work.

Many authors agree that reflective practice is a multidimensional process that seeks to problematise a broad range of professional situations encountered by the practitioner so that they can become potential learning situations (Johns, 1998; Greenwood, 1998; Boyd and Fales, 1983; Schön, 1983). Thus reflection enables a continuation of learning and development in which the practitioner grows in and through their practice (Todd and Freshwater, 1999).

More recently reflective practice has been linked to the emergence of the expert practitioner and advanced nursing practice (Rolfe, 1998a; Johns, 1998; Benner, 1984). While the interpretation of what constitutes the expert practitioner continues to be expanded and refined, what is clear is that the practitioner with 'conscious expertise' is one who has a willingness to reflect, is willing to learn from experience, is open-minded and does not function in isolation (Dewey, 1933). These are attributes that are closely aligned with the reflective practitioner (Schön, 1983) and incidentally the fundamental characteristics underpinning clinical governance (DoH, 1999b). Much of the literature identifies that the practitioner, when engaged in the process of reflection, travels through three distinct stages, namely those of reflection, criticism and action (Atkins and Murphy, 1993; Schön, 1983; van Manen, 1977). During this process the practitioner creates a space within which to view their espoused theories, beliefs and values alongside their theories in action with the intent of uncovering contradictions. As the practitioner becomes more aware of their own 'guiding fictions' so the possibility of choice, intentionality and deliberative nursing practice becomes more of a reality. McLeod (1996) explicates this move to intentional practice succinctly,

The possibility of choice arises from reflexivity, since the person does not respond automatically to events but acts intentionally based on awareness of alternatives.

An area that continues to be debated is that of the facilitation of reflective practice. Just as practice cannot be changed in isolation, it is argued that practitioners struggle to objectify their own beliefs, values and actions without the benefit of another perspective. Clinical supervision, also linked with practice development (UKCC, 1996a), appears to be the ideal forum within which to foster reflective practice, although some authors have questioned whether or not reflective practice needs to be an integral part of clinical supervision (Fowler and Chevannes, 1998). This chapter is based on the assumption that effective reflective practice always requires guidance of some sort and is both an internal and external activity. The role of clinical supervision in practice development is addressed in more detail in *Section Three* of this book.

The role of reflection in practice development

It is largely agreed that practice development nurses act as experts, providing guidance on the development and implementation of best practice, supporting innovation and change, and encouraging professional development (Glover, 1998). Few would disagree that practice development requires that practitioners have opportunities to critically appraise their work (and that of others) in order to ensure that practice is evidence-based.

Reflection on and in practice represents a parallel process to practice development and provides an opportunity for doing just this.

Reflective practice can be seen as a companion and pre-cursor to practice development in many ways. Not only does it help to assess if behaviour is congruent with espoused values and beliefs, it also assists in the development of autonomy through self-monitoring (Freshwater, 1998). In addition it can prevent complacency in everyday practice, which it has been argued, risks becoming routinised (Walsh and Ford, 1989). As previously mentioned, with effective reflection practice becomes more conscious, deliberative and intentional, and nursing practice moves closer towards seamless care as practitioners are encouraged to develop an understanding of complex situations involving other disciplines.

Table 4.1: Model of reflection for practice development (Freshwater, 1998)

Level of reflection	Model of reflection	Stage of development
Descriptive	Reflective diaries, reporting incidents. Reflection on action	Practice becomes conscious
Dialogic	Discourse with peers in various arenas including clinical supervision	Practice becomes deliberative
Critical	Able to provide reasoning for actions by engaging in critical conversation with practice/self/others	Transformation of practice/practice development/ innovation

Furthermore, reflection on beliefs, values and norms offers the opportunity to examine, articulate and generate local philosophies and theories of care, as well as assessing the contribution that individual units make to health care delivery at a national level. The generation and assessment of informal theory is something that is inherent in both the process of reflection and the development of practice.

Practice as theory generating

Human action is never theoretical or accidental, even if the theory involved is implicit or tacit (Arygris and Schön, 1974). Models of reflection provide a way of redeeming theories in use which may be tacit (Greenwood, 1998). Emphasising the importance of theorising about knowledge grounded in practice, it represents a dialectic between knowing and doing (Lumby, 1998), regarding practice as a form of knowing (Benner, 1984). Unfortunately, the experiential knowledge embedded in everyday practice, and embodied in the subsequent practice narratives, is still judged using scientific measures and is caught in a competitive dialogue with empirical knowledge.

This does little to progress the development of reflective strategies as Lumby (1998) points out,

Reflection as a research tool or method continues to be perceived as questionable as far as issues of validity, reliability and generalisation are concerned, often forcing nurses to abandon such strategies or to manipulate them in a way which ensures loss of integrity.

This results in evidence-based practice, reflection and practice development becoming dichotomised and reminiscent of the theory-practice gap.

The interface between research, practice and theory has a long history of being problematic (Freshwater, 1998; Rolfe, 1996; Kitson *et al*, 1996). For practice to be evidence-based each individual nurse needs not only to be aware of their own hypotheses and theories, but also to reflect on them in action. This enables the practitioner to test them and modify their actions.

The focus of practice development is the patient and quality of care which is measured against standards of good practice (Coombs and Holgate, 1998). Criticisms of reflective practice focus mainly on its failure to demonstrate its usefulness (evidence of improved practice) through research studies. Day (1993), for example, argues that how reflection changes practice is unknown. The positivist voice is present in these criticisms, which ignore the focus of reflective practice as a starting point in favour of a defining point, although this is understandable in the current climate of evidence-based practice. This chapter proposes that reflection is a research method and that evidence of best practice can be accessed through reflexive strategies. However, the evidence needs to be measured using the appropriate framework. It is not fitting to measure a subjective experience using strategies akin to the positivist paradigm. This demonstrates a lack of understanding not only of reflection, but also of the process of nursing.

Reflection, like some areas of practice development, has developed its own estimation of rigour, this can be referred to as critical subjectivity (Heron, 1998). In order for critical subjectivity to be integral to everyday practice there are a number of prerequisites. One such requirement is that of developing a practicum, that is an environment that is conducive to learning. A suitable work base for establishment of critical reflectivity is one that encourages reflection and is committed to the development of professional practice; every individual is engaged in collaborative inquiry and dialogue as co-subjects and co-researchers, with everyone consciously trying to develop their practice.

Summary

Reflective practice is a powerful tool, which enables nurses to begin to challenge established practice. However, reflection is not just about gaining access to individual contradictions in values and beliefs through retrospection, it is also about transforming practice (Freshwater, 1998). Practice development is also about transformation, but of what? The practitioner, the profession or practice or of all three? When nursing practice is changed through reflection the practitioner is also transformed, for one is inextricably linked to the other.

Nursing practice and its complexities acquire meaning through reflection in the telling of the practice narrative. In addition, awareness of one's own story and one's own part in practice, has a necessary corollary, that is the voice and story of the other, the patient (Skultans, 1998).

In order to develop a knowledge base for practice development, it is necessary to combine formal and informal knowledge and theory. Reflection achieves this moving between the boundaries of research, education and practice. Further, when engaged in the act of reflection, the practitioner is engaged in a process of critical subjectivity, that is consciousness in the midst of action (Heron, 1998). Critical subjectivity celebrates primary subjective experience, accepting that experiential articulation of being in the world of practice is the ground of all knowing.

It is argued that practice development needs to occur in an environment that is conducive to learning, one that encourages reflection, in which every individual is consciously trying to develop their nursing practice.

5

Hospital-based practice development

Lee Beresford

Having worked as a practice development nurse for the last four years, I have many times been asked, 'What is practice development? What is it about?' Taking a literal stance, one could say that 'development' is concerned with becoming larger, fuller, or more mature or organised; and that 'practice' can be seen as action as opposed to theory. Sounds simple enough, doesn't it? That is of course true, if one assumes an uncomplicated relationship between the 'action' of practice, or those who practice, and the 'organisation' of development.

What is hospital-based practice development like? To answer this question it is necessary to ask, 'what is the difference between institutional settings and anywhere else?' Apart from the obvious geographical ones, the main difference is cultural. Groups are bound by common beliefs and expectations and conforming to common rules. Hospitals and hospital departments, for example wards, have these like any other situation where human beings gather together for protracted periods of time with a purpose in mind. Although it is important to recognise and respect differences and to not try to reduce many views to just one view, extreme cultural forms such as 'tribalism' are almost always a hindrance to programmes of practice development, and should be guarded against at all times through raised awareness.

It is commonly argued that in institutional settings one is perhaps more likely to encounter change-resistant personalities and structures. However, the reliability of this charge is far from clear. It seems believable that there has been less investment in ward-based nurses' development than their colleagues' in the community (NPDN, 1999). Yet, paradoxically, hospital-based services often lead the way in new developments in health care provision including nursing (Page, 1995; Kitson and Currie, 1996).

How is it done? There is no one answer to this question. Effective and lasting practice development is likely to follow the stages outlined below, which can be seen as an iterative process:

Stage 1: change thinking (the people).

Stage 2: change structures (the rules).

Stage 3: change practice (the experience).

Wright (1996) suggests that personal development is a necessary precondition of practice development. To change one's ways of thinking is an intensely personal (ideally developmental) experience. In a sense, Wright is arguing for the position that all practice development begins with the self. If one regards the first stage of personal development as, 'opening up personal thinking', and accepting the need for change in one's own practice, then this is indeed a truism.

In practice development there are strong arguments for accepting that it is 'thought, attitude, and perception' behind practice that has to develop first. Such progress, if correctly stimulated and guided, will lead initially to an increased ability to challenge own-practice, and then to accept challenges from others in a constructive dialogue, thus developing a strategy-forming outlook (strategic thinking). In order to do this effectively one must first assess the 'development readiness' of the team or teams that are to be worked with. This assessment can be achieved by means of an immersion in the team, that is, through working shifts, attending team meetings, building relationships with the team as though one were an ordinary new member of the team.

The purpose of such an assessment is to identify a baseline position on the following: current staff issues and concerns; local political influences and the 'grape-vine' (who talks to whom, how often, and where); the degree of 'free' thinking and ideation present in the workforce. These can be regarded as a measurement of the vigour of any team. The assessor should seek out and woo 'opinion leaders', those who can carry forward an idea or a vision within a team but do not necessarily have position power. He or she should work to develop within themselves the embodiment of a balanced understanding, a real feel for the overall position of the team. This process undeniably requires a significant degree of confidence and skill. It can be personally challenging for any individual who may wish to attempt it. Staff can be unforgiving, suspicious, and obstructive. Strength of commitment and vision, however, will help those intent upon being the spark that lights the fires of practice development to succeed.

An alternative method of team assessment is suggested by Anderson and West (1994). The Team Climate Inventory (TCI) is a questionnaire assessment tool in which staff are invited to record their strength of agreement or disagreement against forty-four Likert-scaled statements. It focuses on communication, innovation, objectives and task styles in any group of professional workers. Walsh and Walsh (1998) have recently researched the efficacy of the Team Climate Inventory on a group of thirty-three ward-based nurses. They concluded that the tool was both easy to administer, and simple to analyse. They claim an accuracy for prediction of team readiness for practice development initiatives, recommending its use to all those involved in practice development.

Although this sounds encouraging and offers the opportunity to appear more 'scientific' and more 'objective' in making an assessment, one must be aware of the limitations of questionnaire-based returns.

Whatever the method of assessment, in order to begin to change thinking and subsequent attitude and perception in individuals within a team, one must engage those individuals 'face to face' and 'on their own ground'. Any opportunity to persuade, influence, sell, argue for a new vision must not be missed. Success in practice development will depend on the establishment of simultaneous changes in team structures, such as team-working patterns, or the (internal and external) communication network. These will reinforce new thinking, and legislate against the resurgence of 'old' practices.

Nurses have long grappled with the challenges caused by poor team working and low morale. It is recognised that practice development is every nurse's business (Page, 1995; Kitson and Currie, 1996: Wright, 1996), but that as with so much in life it is perhaps best achieved with the help of others. Practice development, and in particular practice development nurses, have risen recently as a force to take up these and other challenges laid before the nursing profession.

Practice development is crucially underpinned by effective team-working structures. Wards and other hospital departments are ready-formed homogenous groups and benefit from many pre-existing factors that will assist the building of team-working. Among the factors that can be considered to contribute to effective team-working are:

- high morale and open channels of communication
- effective conflict resolution strategies
- a feeling that each individual matters and will be supported by others
- investment in personal development

- common goals and a sense of working together
- feeling safe to suggest new ideas
- a bottom-up inclusive approach.

Walsh and Walsh, 1998

Getting functioning communication structures right is the most important aspect of any practice development initiative. A network, or web, must be constructed that is able to supply the needs of all members of the team, from the lowest grades up, and the needs of the organisation in which the initiative takes place. An example communication network from a programme of practice development (Beresford, 1998) is shown in *Figure 5.1.*

Figure 5.1: Communication chart

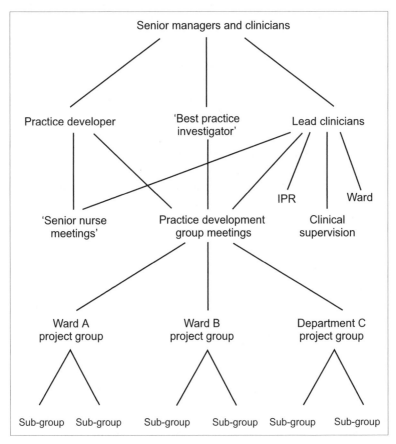

Naming the initiative is often a helpful strategy. Create a 'catchy' title that has some relation to the work you are undertaking. Commonly these are taken from things people say when describing their concerns or defining the issues for example 'lumpy mashed potatoes' or 'the odd sock'. Alternatively, they can be designed to inspire, 'To infinity... and beyond!' Both can be subtitled with a more explanatory line. On a serious note, publicising, advertising or touting your initiative is of the utmost importance, and your communication strategy should include presentations in a wide range of media.

Documents will need to be produced at an early stage. These should include; introductory texts, newsletters, minutes of meetings, flyers, posters etc. Always use the 'catchy' title, and if possible develop a recognisable logo. Branding your concept will inevitably help with selling it. These communiqués will need to say the same thing, but in different 'languages'. The target audience may be wide, from CEO to nursing assistant. The documents can say many things to persuade, assuage or inspire the individual reader. The message at whatever level it is aimed, should aim to answer the question, 'what's in it for me?'

An example of a question and answer format (designed in this instance for a nursing audience) is illustrated below (Beresford, 1998):

Why do we need to work together?

Wards A, B, and Department C share many aspects of nursing philosophy, knowledge and practice. There is much that can be learned from each other, as well as from the process of learning together. An old adage says 'many hands make light work', and in this case combining our efforts will help us to achieve improvement in our service whilst maintaining a full attention to our day-to-day duties.

What does all this mean for me?

As a member of staff working within the three departments you will find several potential benefits from the successful completion of the programme. Among these perhaps the most important is the opportunity to develop as an individual, with a greater clarity of role and clearer, relevant, and stimulating objectives, thus enabling you to personally contribute in a way that influences the longer-term development of the service at many different levels. This will increase both your own and your colleagues' sense of job satisfaction. Interesting and stimulating opportunities are worth having in your work. It will also help us to recruit new nurses to the wards, and to attract more resources to assist in the continuing need to improve patient care.

I want to be involved. How can I do this?
Everyone can play a part in developing the service we provide. Grade and experience (or lack of it) are no barriers to your involvement. Everyone will have the opportunity to contribute in some way. You may wish to join one of the groups that will be set up in forming the framework for the programme. You are encouraged to harness your enthusiasm, interest, ideas, and pride in nursing to improve your and your colleagues' ability to identify areas of nursing work for investigation/improvement, to work to change your practice in an effort to provide a continually improving quality service. You are encouraged to speak to your department leader, who will welcome any suggestion you may have, and be happy to support your participation in this programme.

The essence of practice development as an activity in any health care setting is multi-disciplinary. However, health service professionals, including nurses, in hospital bases are often accused of being less than enthusiastic supporters of the idea of working toward a multi-disciplinary future vision. There are many potential reasons for this: a limited level of exposure to the multi-disciplinary team; closed mind set; closeness of the team; traditional ways of behaving; just getting on with the job; suspiciousness. Hospital-based departments, such as wards, are areas of focused nursing activity. Often this activity is intensely focused. This kind of working environment can lead to the development of a single-mindedness of purpose that can be difficult to divert.

As previously stated, setting up effective communication systems within and across teams to 'get people talking' is essential in introducing any subject for development. This introduction is important in that it affords an opportunity to gradually become aware of, and to explore, a subject without too much of a feeling of pressure. Rail-roading is certainly not conducive to practice development. Soon, however, there becomes the need to 'get people doing'. A big stumbling block to this with large groups or teams may often be a lack of specific skills or knowledge. This first hurdle could be your last if you are not prepared to embark upon a team-wide course of training. It is certainly true that training can be expensive but costs can be reduced significantly. In-house training may be the answer.

Look around, the expertise is often locally available. Senior members of the team can become workshop leaders if shown how to organise and present their material. Training within any practice development programme is often best undertaken with teams than individuals because members develop shared goals, and can support each other in the improvement of their practice (Kitwood, 1997). Workshop formats are informal, yet allow staff to learn, shape, and be actively involved in their own development (Hanily, 1995).

In changing practice, whether it be your own or that of others, innovation, the bringing forth of new ideas is an important component. However, the management of change in nursing is a process that is undeniably fraught with difficulty. If poorly approached and handled, it may stifle emergent innovation, and may also deter nurses from sharing their ideas. Equally, nurses may suffer from 'innovation fatigue' the result of over exposure to stimulation without substantive and satisfying resolution. Practice development requires change in an NHS culture resistant to change (Walsh and Walsh, 1998). For a team of nurses or any other clinicians to be innovative, it is essential that the management of that workforce commits to, and clearly demonstrates, a participatory and collaborative style.

Generally, quality assurance is viewed as a way of protecting the needs and interests of clients, and of satisfying inspectors and managers that basic standards of care are being met. Kitwood (1997), however, suggests that the whole process has another function,

> *... it is a way of giving systematic feedback to staff, and hence, if handled correctly, of giving them assurance in their work.*

Data from research and audit should be made available to staff as a basis for discussion. This is so ideas can be considered and new ones stimulated and that plans can be devised for the localised improvement of care. To do this is to set up a development loop, a sort of virtuous circle of advancement.

In summary, practice development can be seen as the driver to research, audit, and clinical effectiveness. It is the medium by which the elements of self and clinical governance are best delivered to nurses and other clinical staff. Practice development should be ultimately regarded as being primarily concerned with the empowerment of staff, and those in their care.

6

Community-based practice development

Andrew Clark

The development of practice for community staff shares some but not all of the problems outlined in the previous chapter and additionally possesses different problems related to diversity and geography.

One distinct advantage when considering group development of community staff in a particular location is the ability to provide cover on an 'emergency only' basis from the next door 'patch' staff or clinic, sliding routine work along to the next available slot. This ability is of course shared by day hospitals who, unlike a ward-based service, can close completely for a day's training if required.

Conversely, geographic base problems make for their own set of unique difficulties with split responsibilities often on different sites, increasing demands on staff coupled with the diverse nature of the skills required to operate in a community environment.

The structure of community staff has changed over the years. Community teams traditionally were staffed by experienced practitioners whose continuing development needs differed from the average ward environment staff, who were often less experienced and more junior in grade. However, it is now common to find community teams whose structure will contain all grades (or at least a proportion thereof) and training needs will reflect accordingly. Increasingly community teams have a large percentage of non registered staff whose needs are often neglected.

A training course designed to implement clinical supervision in a community team for instance can be achieved with 'one hit'. As most work can be planned the entire team can be taken out of the service provision for a day with cover from neighbouring areas. The advantages are obvious. Every one hears the same message at the same time and initiatives can be introduced in a shorter space of time. The same approach cannot be used in the in-patient environment (ward) where several courses accommodating days off and 24-hour ward cover would be required to achieve the same level of message infiltration in the same percentage of staff .

There would appear to be three main strands of continuing education. Firstly, the mandatory study days covering the kinds of subjects everyone loves to hate from basic life support to the dreaded fire lecture, health and safety, moving and handling, infection control and so on. Next are those training events designed to improve your knowledge of your speciality with a short to medium term gain in knowledge and skills. ENB courses in your specialty, for example, or clinical supervision training or learning a new technical skill would be good illustrations of this.

Lastly, there are the long term long courses designed to improve your own wider knowledge and only influence and benefit the organisation in the longer term by having staff trained to a higher level. These would include various degree and diploma courses up to Master and PhD level.

Every member of staff has to attend those in the first group. Unfortunately there are all too often complaints from staff nurses about mandatory in-service education programmes, stating that they are repetitious, time-consuming, often too basic and, at times, downright boring (Henry, 1997). In the world of adult education where the learners have complex expectations, the educator must make an extra effort to meet the customers' (learners') needs (Clark, 1999).

Obtaining study leave is becoming more difficult for clinical nurses in the current economic climate, but the need to develop new clinical skills and to maintain existing good practice remains of prime importance to patient care (Gould and Chamberlain, 1997). Historically business ethics in the health care industry and continuing education specifically, has created little or no problems. Individuals within organisations/agencies provided whatever continuing education was considered necessary at little or no cost to the consumer. However, as monies became scarce for institutions, many became less willing to provide education for little or no income. Simultaneously, it was realised that continuing education for health professionals could generate significant monies so many entrepreneurial persons entered the field for profit (Pearson, 1987). This has led to the need for an individual or institution to be more selective than in the past when spending hard earned cash on training events and facilitators for staff.

There is now of course a mandatory element to training with the advent of post registration education and practice (PREP) (UKCC, 1995b). However the literature shows a fragmented, inequitable and poorly funded provision of continuing professional education to date in the UK (Furze and Pearcey, 1999).

Unlike many commercial companies who are able to have a single vision, the NHS is unique among organisations. It has many layers with different visions, many agendas and a multitude of professional staff groups, each dedicated to advancing their own particular set of objectives while purporting to enhance the quality of patient care.

Community staff have much to be concerned with. Recent media attention has focused on mental health care in a far from positive manner for example, and evidence suggests that the care programme approach has not proved a total success (North *et al*, 1993).

Despite this, it remains the foundation on which a series of policy directives has been based over the last 5 years, and it is difficult to disagree with the fundamental philosophy, which reflects the basic principles underpinning the delivery of effective mental health care in the community (Sullivan, 1997). Additionally the introduction of the Mental Health (Patients in the Community) Act 1995 has been the cause of much concern, although there has been little published debate from nurses or community psychiatric nurses (CPNs) (Coffey, 1997).

All community staff await with some trepidation the effect of the new primary care groups and the full effect of clinical governance. If fully implemented, clinical governance will be the major force in long term change in all aspects of provision of health care services in the UK. The search for evidence-based practice and the use of research to enhance care continues with perhaps more pace than ever.

This leaves us with a dilemma. Many nurses still feel somewhat ill equipped to critically analyse research. Yet one of the main rudiments of practice development is that it is concerned with promoting evidence-based practice and creating stronger partnerships between practice and research (Cutcliffe *et al*, 1998). It is therefore essential to be able to dissect evidence in order to discover what is good research and good evidence on which to base the development of practice.

Unfortunately research findings do not usually come in neat, consistent, ready to use or even easy to find packages. Nurses are often surprised to find when they review articles that there is in fact a preponderance of them that are not research-based (Strickland and Fishman, 1994). Yet there is much hope as many university-based continuing education and ENB courses contain modules designed to assist the current/next generation of nurses with research appreciation and interpretation.

Although ongoing education is an expectation of all nurses in today's climate of increasing technology and patient acuity, little is known about the attitudes, beliefs, and values of the general staff nurse toward on-the-job learning (White *et al*, 1998). However, it is clear that in order to ensure optimum professional competence in meeting the health care needs of society, continuous updating of nursing education is required. While professional competence is a personal responsibility, organised systems are necessary as facilitators (Crapanzano, 1999).

Brooks and Fletcher (1998) suggested in their study of advanced practice nurses that there were three major needs identified:

1. Enhancement of clinical practice skills and knowledge in specialty areas.
2. Education about future changes in the advanced practice nurse (APN) role (this is an American reference which equates roughly to our nurse practitioner level).
3. Education in management strategies for the changing health care delivery system.

There is every reason to think that other community staff, regardless of speciality, also share these concerns.

It is clear that nursing staff development programmes must be responsive to current changes in health care (Goodman, 1997). Yet staff have 'change fatigue' and care must be taken when launching new initiatives lest they appear to be the flavour of the month and therefore rejected before they have been given a chance to flourish. The internal market damaged much co-operation and some organisations have yet to recover from the drive for efficiency and value of the 1980s which took the view that if there was no perceivable immediate benefit to patients there was no place for that initiative or service (Johnson and Scholes, 1993). Indeed, changes in the delivery of health care have created an environment viewed as uncaring to both the patient and health care providers. Thus, teaching concepts of health and caring becomes a priority for nurse educators (Gramling and Nugent, 1998).

As a consequence of this, continuing education in some sectors has been stretched to a point where demand will outstrip supply by a significant factor. The net effect is a drift to alternative providers and damage to morale and staff retention, as staff, feeling that the organisation cares little for them move to areas which will provide more adequate levels of training. Additionally the difficulties students experience in applying theory to practice are well documented and educationalists have employed a variety of techniques in an effort to enhance effective application (Phillips *et al*, 1998). They must continue to strive to develop new methods of facilitation to hold the interest of the 'student' who has many other pressures on her time both professionally and personally. The most formidable task facing an educator is the planning and development of new activities. When the target audience consists of experienced professional adults, the challenge is even greater, since these learners require a special understanding and faculty with effective teaching habits (Crapanzano, 1999). Proper regard must be given to the wealth of knowledge that these experienced professionals bring to the classroom.

As we enter the twenty-first century health services are confronted with many of the same challenges facing other organisations. These include restructuring to increase competitiveness and providing services more efficiently with smaller staff (Helgerson, 1992). These challenges will undoubtedly impact both directly and indirectly on practice development (Stern, 1992). There is little doubt that this impact is set to continue.

7

The development of the consultant nurse

James Dooher

The emergence of practice development nurses (PDNs) and their development into the role of consultants can be traced back to 1988 when the Nurses and Midwives Pay Review Body introduced clinical grading. Clinical grading was designed to identify and differentiate between the responsibility and skills required for different posts. It also stipulated that at every level of the nursing hierarchy there should be one responsible individual. This had the effect of bringing into focus the role of clinical nurses, and at the same time began to place traditional nurse managers at risk. Their role was immediately placed in jeopardy as nurses of grade 'F' and above assumed the authority appropriate to their grade.

This dramatic erosion of nurse managers' responsibilities led to many taking early retirement and the re-configuration of clinical services. Employers perhaps saw the opportunity to reduce costs further, by devolving the power base and increasing the responsibilities of clinical based staff. The role of 'G' grades was seen as pivotal at this time, and many lost their title of sister/charge nurse to become ward managers. The issue of accountability was reiterated to all nurses, together with a renewed focus upon the legal and moral obligations of each clinical grade. The roles and responsibilities of the ward manager often generated competing and incompatible demands between the clinical and managerial agendas, producing new dilemmas for both the individuals in post, and their employers. Management in the health care sector became increasingly divergent with the introduction of the general manager. The traditional nurse management role was increasingly seen as a gravy train, ineffective, and diverting resources away from the bedside. Costs needed to be seen to be reducing and often employers in the shape of Health Authorities and the new 'Trusts' re-shuffled the human resource to appease this view. Management costs were cut through a process of natural attrition, new clinical titles retaining many of the old function and the introduction of practice development nurses to carry on an old role under a new clinical guise.

The development of practice development nurses and clinical nurse specialists (CNS) was inconsistent in terms of both role and responsibility. The generalist practice development nurse was often given a 'G or H' grade whereas the previous nurse manager retired on an 'I' with the same job description. The clinical nurse specialist on the other hand, was seen as an expert in their field with a very narrow focus, and consequently a much rarer breed. The scope of the clinical nurse specialist's role broadly replicated that of their counterparts in the United States, with advanced practice skills being the primary focus. Research, education and being seen as a role model made up the rest of their function. Scott (1999) identified the most common advanced practice skills associated with clinical nurse specialists, which included areas such as psychotherapy, family therapy, grief therapy, pain and wound management, crisis intervention and advanced assessments together with pharmacological and surgical interventions.

In the UK, the *Health of the Nation* (DoH, 1992a) White Paper identified breast cancer, skin cancer and health promotion as examples of specialist themes. On the other hand, practice development nurses appeared to have inherited a much more generic role which included many of the tasks and responsibilities bequeathed by the demise of the old nurse manager. These included responsibilities for audit rather than research, investigations of poor practice, mandatory training rather than education and the administration and responsibility for budgets. This placed PDNs in the no man's land between management and clinical practice, a position that ultimately undermined their effectiveness and their perceived value to both camps. This change was initiated and sustained for just over ten years by means of continual reorganisation and displacement of nurse managers.

The introduction of what has been described as a 'Super Nurse' or nurse consultant was met with a mixed response. An editorial in the *Nursing Times* (1999) headlined the 'muddled thinking and dodgy arithmetic' behind the Government's plan to initiate this new grade, said to have both the status and pay of their medical counterparts. The posts were proposed to provide an alternative career path to management where post holders could still retain patient contact, combining expert practice, leadership and research. The title consultant nurse seems rather contradictory too, in that after years of nurses divesting themselves of medical models it has been directly lifted from consultant medical model (Monkman and Hempstead, 1999); or worse from the profit driven world of commercial consultancy, where short-term fixes are delivered by sharp suited 'experts'. Stephen (1999) suggested that applicants would need to satisfy the UKCC standards for higher practice with their academic profile demonstrating at least Masters level if not clinical doctorate attainment.

Clearly good nursing leadership will require more than just an academic ability and Yates (1999) considers that there are four Es that constitute a successful leader:

1. **Envisioner**: having a clear view of what is to be achieved.
2. **Enabler**: supporting the development of stakeholders and providing the right tools to achieve their vision.
3. **Energiser**: charismatic enthusiasm which motivates people to act and achieve success.
4. **Empowerer**: providing an atmosphere where leaders and followers are mutually accountable for the achievement of their jointly owned vision.

To achieve a creative, dynamic, proactive and sustainable place in the health care system, consultant nurses will need to be both credible and robust. They will need to be able to persuade colleagues to embrace their agenda through the power of expertise rather than the power of management. They will need to demonstrate leadership from within rather than the margins, and they will need to motivate their nursing and multi-disciplinary co-workers providing a convincing line of reasoning for the value of their individual and collective agendas.

If the optimistic figures predicted by England's outgoing Chief Nurse Yvonne Moores (1999) are to be believed, then a significant increase in funding for both pay and education is required. She suggests that by 2002 we may expect to see 200–300 consultant nurses who spend at least 50% of their time in clinical practice. Frank Dobson (the ex-Secretary of State for Health) mooted the number would be nearer 5000. In January 2000, 141 posts were announced with the current Secretary of State for Health, Alan Milburn, suggesting that the glass ceiling had been removed and the barriers to optimise the potential for the very best nurses had been broken down (Munro, 2000). Understandably, the new Chief Nurse Sarah Mullally was gushing in her praise for the announcement. She stated that,

> ... *these new posts create a significant new career opportunity to retain the most experienced and expert nurses, midwives and health visitors in the NHS, doing what they came into the profession to do.*

Her optimism raged on as she pronounced that,

... these appointments mean better care and treatment and improved care for patients and communities.

Munro, 2000

Clearly great things are expected from these posts. Pay levels are predicted to commence at around £27,460 rising to £42,010. This is the first blow to consultant nurses being attributed equitable status to their medical counterparts, whose starting salaries average £47,000. The second factor which undermines parity relates to the academic rigour of pre and post registration education. In an interview with *Nursing Management*, Tony Butterworth (1999) suggested that some Universities offering nursing for the first time saw the opportunity to increase volume by 30% but 'did not become sufficiently attentive to the niceties of the subject'. Considering that basic medical training involves a six-year programme as opposed to nursing's three years, and subject reviews to assess quality and standards in nurse education are still in their infancy, it is legitimate to draw a conclusion that pre registration nurse education falls short of the academic rigour one might expect to offer clear comparisons. This is further compromised with the disparity of entrance criteria to professional training. Nursing is widening the entry gate and allowing an increasing range of vocational qualifications and even exemption through accreditation of prior learning both experiential and academic, to prospective students. This does nothing to uphold the public's or the profession's perception of itself.

The agenda set out in a range of government reports including; *New NHS Modern and Dependable* (DoH, 1997), *Making a Difference* (DoH, 1999a), *Saving lives our healthier nation* (DoH, 1999c) represents the targets from which the impact of consultant nurses will be calculated. Yet as the community is carved up into primary care trusts and the in-patient sector is being increasingly driven by efficiency savings, there may be an inevitable shift to utilise the skill base of consultant nurses to cut costs rather than improve quality. It is felt by many that consultant nurses will become the scapegoats of the both the nursing profession and the NHS at large. It has been suggested that if the government were really committed to the idea it would have created thousands of posts, perhaps one for every fifty nurses, rather than at best a couple of hundred.

Consultant nurses will be rare enough to be professionally isolated and embarrassed by their relatively large salaries, making them easy targets for criticism. The added pressure of continually justifying the position and the salary it attracts will further marginalise the role leading to occupational stress. Payne and Firth-Couzens (1987) suggested that a job can be demanding without causing stress if the worker is well supported. It is doubtful that consultant nurses will feel supported, rather the opposite, leading to increased pressure, reduced performance and ultimately the antithesis of the reason for their existence. In these times of financial hardship with year on year savings, consultant nurses will be perceived as the 'fat cats' of the profession and are doomed to fail. It is anticipated that consultant nurses will attempt to offer peer support to each other with perhaps the formulation of a national forum. Of course this will require regular meetings, regional representatives and organisation. If 50% of the role is intended to be spent in clinical practice, then these additional supportive aspects will erode research, education and the strategic development time nursing so badly needs. It will be the clinical time that is actually eroded due to its relatively low profile and status, and the consultant nurses need to publicly justify their position through high profile activity. The optimism espoused by the chief nurse is misplaced. These roles will not save nursing, the NHS or the government. They are a quick fix, designed for sound bite politics. Consultant nurses will focus on the most rewarding and visible areas of their speciality out of a need for self-preservation, and the non-clinical demands of their role will prove too attractive to resist.

Further evidence of this flawed scheme can be seen through the applicability and relevance to the independent sector. Despite the fact that the independent sector employs over 550,000 staff (Shepherd,1999) there does not seem to be any element of the strategy to embrace this very important aspect of health delivery. Shepherd goes on to suggest that 25% of all nurses on the UKCC register work outside the NHS. If this is the case, then the question of how consultant nurses may offer leadership to this often self-employed disparate group of professionals is one that remains unanswered for the foreseeable future.

It may be said that the consultant nurse role will never live up to expectations. If prospective candidates really are 'Super Nurses' they will be able to see through the rhetoric and recognise that it is flawed to the core, and investment, kudos and acknowledgement would have been far more effective if it rewarded the thousands of nurses with twenty-four hour responsibility for care rather than its creation of a class divide within the nursing profession.

8

The organisation and management of practice development

Andrew Clark

There is no one structure which will provide an ideal solution to the problems of how to organise practice development staff. This will very much depend on the organisational relationships that are required by the ward team, department, area trust or unit, and also the tasks that they are expected to perform. Indeed, there is evidence to suggest that organisations should experiment as there are no clear rules as to how hospitals or other trusts should be broken down (White, 1993). Therefore one model of practice development is not recommended over another.

The ideal solution is to first have an overview of some of the models provided; then analyse the tasks and desired outcomes of the practice development staff and the needs of your organisation before designing a structure.

In reality few of us have this luxury. However a few moments examining how others have arranged the practice development function and the annotated comments of the authors may well pay dividends if you are tasked with setting up a practice development service. Additionally, you may well glean examples of good practice which will fit your service rather than having to re-invent the practice development wheel.

In many cases the relationship to the management function will have a decisive effect on the organisational structure which is adopted.

Historically few, if any, health service structures have been created with a specific purpose in mind; often they have been adapted from existing services and tailored to fit regardless. If practice development fails because of poor organisational design, it is not the fault of the practice developers, rather it is the fault of those that designed the organisational relationships. These relationships are key to the success of practice development projects and attention should be paid in the early stages to ensure the correct model base is chosen.

The following are some examples of the way practice development is organised:

- centralised department of practice development or clinical excellence staffed by full-time or a mixture of full-time and part-time assigned staff
- project based practice development facilitated by full-time or part PD staff
- directorate based PD staff informally linked to a central department, eg. Department of Practice Development or Nursing and Quality/Clinical Excellence.

PD staff directly accountable to managers are found in some services, although there are problems as the practice development agenda is almost always compromised by the management agenda which appears to take precedence.

Figure 8.1: Centrally based practice development function with specialty/directorate links

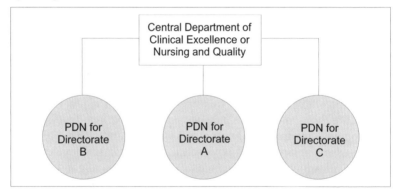

This model with a centrally based department (commonly called Nursing and Quality or Department of Clinical Excellence), with staff lent out to various specialities or directorates, has a number of advantages for the practice development staff. They can share expertise and provide support and supervision for each other and this model reduces the sense of isolation which many practice development staff feel. It also provides a greater pool of resources and expertise to use on practice development projects.

It has a further advantage that strategic projects are more easily co-ordinated and less likely to be laid to one side by the directorate staff.

There are disadvantages: directorate management may feel that they have little control over the function of the practice development staff and the inevitable conflict of agendas that this brings. Also, there is a possibility of resistance to the centre from the outlying directorates who may not wish their agenda to be set centrally.

The directorate structure which originated in the USA has been somewhat slavishly followed with little evaluation of efficacy. It can be described as 'a sub unit led by a Clinical Director who is accountable for the directorates functioning' (Capewell, 1992). However, there is a tendency for competition and isolation to rear its head and there is often duplication of effort due to communication deficits.

Figure 8.2: Specialty or directorate based staff with links to central function

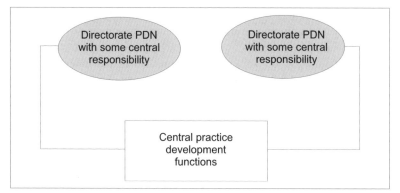

This model has the advantage for directorate management in that they perceive that they have a greater degree of control over the role of 'their' practice development staff. (This may or not be the case.) It also allows a more localised focus for staff development and the feeling that you 'belong somewhere' which in large organisations may well be of some importance.

However it makes the co-ordination of strategic and trust wide projects difficult if the practice development staff are managed by different parts of the organisation with competing priorities and agendas. The practice development staff can feel torn between demands on their time from the local directorate/speciality and the central department. Project-based practice development is covered in *Chapter 11, p.91.*

Should practice development staff have a full-time or part-time role?

Some services use staff on a part-time basis where part of their role is ward or department-based and part of their role is practice development. (This may or may not involve an increase in remuneration for the practice development part of the role.) It is argued that keeping staff in their main role with a part-time practice development function has benefits in terms of allowing fully clinically based staff to influence practice development. In reality there is always a conflict of interest and demands on their time can lead to a punishing workload. Often the staff member will end up with a dilemma and it is difficult to see the advantages for the staff who are placed in this invidious position, organisations must not make unrealistic demands on staff to effectively cover two jobs for the price of one. In the long term, organisations will lose more than they gain.

Example 1: G grade with part-time practice development nurse, role 1

I accepted the role as I thought that it would benefit not only my career but also give me the opportunity to have a role outside of my immediate area and influence practice in a wider context. The work was exciting and challenging, but in the end the sheer volume of work overtook me. The reality of the allocated hours proved to be very different, I simply ended up doing two jobs, I couldn't really concentrate on anything and my physical and mental health suffered.

Management were unrealistic in what they felt we should achieve in the few hours a week allocated to practice development.

This is not the case for all organisations as some staff successfully combine split roles and great benefit is derived in terms of the individual the organisation and for patient care (see Example 2).

Example 2: G grade with part-time practice development nurse, role 2

I love the variety that the role brings me; I never seem to have two days the same. I move from a meeting to a clinical role and then to an educational activity so I feel very lucky.

I do recognise however that I have a supportive F grade to assist me with my clinical workload and my manager is sympathetic to the demands of the practice development role.

The reality is that practice development should not be practised in isolation, as a development in practice will impinge on the role of other disciplines to a greater or lesser extent. Multi-disciplinary practice development is both desirable for patient care and has many benefits for the staff involved. Most multi-disciplinary teams actually function as networks and joint training and development can be very rewarding and enlightening for all concerned.

Does management have a role in practice development?

It is possible to argue that management functions should be an integral part of the practice development function. It is also equally possible to argue that it should be completely separate from the management function.

There are both advantages and disadvantages to integration and separation of function. It is important to stress that there is not one proven model which will offer a universal solution to the problem of how to organise practice development. The local circumstances will in many cases dictate the starting point. It is however useful to bear in mind two important issues.

Often the difficulties of attaching practice development to the management function are underestimated as is the perception that practice development staff are merely part of management. This is unhelpful for both the practitioners and for the practice development nurse who then expends a deal of time explaining that the next project or initiative is practice development based and not driven by a management agenda which is often alien to the clinical environment. Conversely, attachment to the management function does carry more power and authority if required.

Secondly, although the separation of function brings with it benefits in terms of staff perception and freedom to work with professional issues, all progress has to be achieved by influence and persuasion rather than by management authority. This can result in the practice development nurse being given responsibility and accountability for something over which she has no power and control, which in turn can lead to stressful situations and failure.

There is a requirement for a balance to be achieved in respect of the six key variables: full-time or part-time; directorate or centrally based; management or professionally attached.

A matrix analysis or cost benefit analysis of the perceived advantages and disadvantages should be performed before embarking on organisational change which leads to development of a practice development service. It can be difficult to backtrack and reorganise practice development services so it is important to get it right first time. It can be argued that the reality of any difficulties are less than the perceived problems. Therefore, a view on how others in the organisation (both those involved and those delivering the PDN service) would view such a venture is vital if the organisation is to achieve a satisfactory outcome in the key area of service provision that is practice development.

Section 2:
The reality of practice development

9

The influence of clinical governance on practice development

Cathy McCargow

Introduction

This chapter identifies how clinical governance influences practice development. It summarises key developments in national policy that have a bearing on this issue and considers what kind of practice development the NHS needs before explaining ways in which clinical governance will support practice development. It then raises some of the issues that staff may confront within their organisations when implementing clinical governance and, finally, it offers some practical suggestions for personal and professional development.

Clinical governance — what the papers say

Clinical governance is central to the new agenda for health care and it features in many national policy initiatives.

The new NHS modern – dependable

The new NHS (DoH, 1997) marked a turning point for the NHS. It replaced the internal market with proposals for integrated care based on partnership and driven by performance. The reforms set out a challenging modernisation agenda for the NHS. The document noted that:

> *The speed of change in science and medicine and the potential of modern information and communication systems require the NHS to embrace change. A modern and dependable NHS will capture developments in modern medicine and information technology. It will be built around the needs of people, not of institutions and it will provide prompt reliable care. It will learn from those at the leading edge of good practice and it will make the best available to all.*

Along with its proposals for organisational change, including the establishment of primary care groups and trusts, the Government determined that there should be a new focus on quality. Every NHS organisation was charged with the duty of embracing 'clinical governance' with quality at the core, both of the organisation and of each member of staff as individual professionals. The document also stressed that NHS Trusts would be expected to strengthen the nursing contribution to the running and development of these organisations.

Chief executives were given a new statutory duty for quality of care. They now carry ultimate responsibility for assuring the quality of services provided by their trust and are required to establish and maintain mechanisms that enable the trust board to be confident that standards are being met. These arrangements build on, systematise and strengthen the existing systems of professional self-regulation. The importance of ensuring that the new arrangements engaged clinical staff at ward level was stressed in the White Paper. Trusts must now receive monthly reports on quality and publish an annual report showing what they are doing to assure it. These arrangements were introduced to help rebuild public confidence in the NHS as a public service, accountable to patients, open to the public and shaped by their views.

In summary, for the first time in the history of the NHS, quality and all that it entails is now firmly on the agenda of every NHS organisation.

A First Class Service

A First Class Service (DoH, 1998a) reaffirmed the principle of a national health service that offered consistently high standards across the country:

> *All patients in the national Health Service are entitled to high quality care. This should not depend on geographic accident of where they happen to live.*

This document built on the initial proposals set out in *The new NHS* (DoH, 1997) White Paper and described a range of proposals to support the delivery of more consistent and higher quality patient care, including:

- Arrangements for setting national quality standards, through National Service Frameworks and the National Institute for Clinical Excellence (NICE). NICE will appraise significant new and existing interventions, advise on best practice and issue evidence-based guidance across the NHS. This will help to reduce variations in standards of treatment and care. It is likely that early work will cover some aspects of care where new nursing roles are developing.

- Mechanisms for ensuring local delivery of high-quality clinical services, through clinical governance reinforced by a new statutory duty of quality and supported by programmes of lifelong learning and local delivery of professional self-regulation for all professions.

- Efficient systems for monitoring the delivery of quality standards, in the form of a new statutory Commission for Health Improvement and an NHS Performance Assessment Framework, along with surveys of patient and user experience.

Figure 9.1 is used to illustrate the links between the various elements.

Figure 9.1: Delivering quality standards

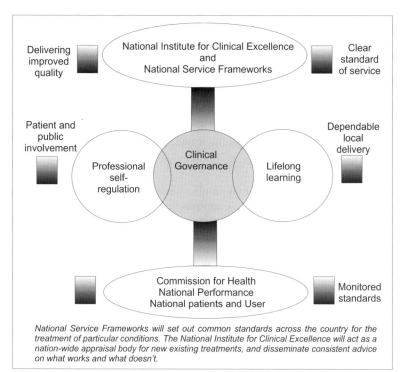

National Service Frameworks will set out common standards across the country for the treatment of particular conditions. The National Institute for Clinical Excellence will act as a nation-wide appraisal body for new existing treatments, and disseminate consistent advice on what works and what doesn't.

Making a Difference

Making a Difference (DoH, 1999a) presents the Government's strategic plans for nursing. It notes that the context of care is changing – changing health and social needs, new technology, rising public expectations and changes within the NHS all pose new challenges. It also acknowledges that nurses, midwives and health visitors are often constrained by structures that limit development and innovation. To strengthen the nursing, midwifery and health visiting contribution, the Government plans to:

+ expand the workforce
+ strengthen education and training
+ develop a modern career framework
+ improve the working lives of nurses, midwives and health visitors
+ help them to contribute to plans to enhance quality
+ strengthen leadership
+ modernise self-regulation
+ encourage new roles and new ways of working.

This will support implementation of clinical governance and put the spotlight on practice development. *Making a Difference* (DoH, 1999a) says that nurses, midwives and health visitors must play a full part in developing National Service Frameworks and clinical governance. Emphasis is placed firmly on improving standards of 'the fundamental and essential aspects of basic care'.

Governance in the New NHS

Governance in the New NHS (DoH, 1999b) describes how financial and organisational assurance is complementary to clinical governance. Controls assurance is described as,

> ... a process designed to provide evidence that NHS organisations are doing their 'reasonable best' to manage themselves so as to meet their objectives and protect patients, staff, and the public and other stakeholders against risks of all kinds... Chief Executives of NHS Trusts and Health Authorities should designate themselves, as accountable officers, or an Executive Director with overall responsibility for ensuring the implementation of controls assurance ...

This is an important circular, in that it acknowledges that clinical excellence does not flourish in a vacuum and that 'getting the organisation right' will increase the likelihood of achieving the desired outcomes for patients. *Figure 9.2* illustrates the links between the different aspects of quality management.

The common thread is risk management, defined as: the culture, processes and structures that are directed towards the effective management of potential opportunities and adverse effects (*Australia/New Zealand Standard*, 1999). To maintain quality, organisations will obviously wish to target resources in a way that addresses serious aspects of risk. It will be important to reduce serious untoward incidents, monitor complaints and legal claims and to take steps to prevent future breakdown in quality.

Equally important is the need to monitor staff sickness, absence and turn-over to identify parts of the organisation that may be in difficulty. The guidance notes that fundamental to the principles of controls assurance is the effective involvement of people to ensure that objectives are met, 'systems make things happen but people make it work'.

Figure 9.2: Controls assurance model

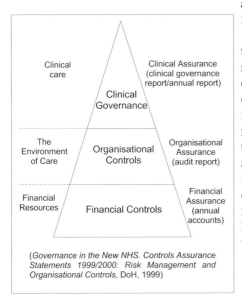

(*Governance in the New NHS. Controls Assurance Statements 1999/2000: Risk Management and Organisational Controls*, DoH, 1999)

What kind of practice development does the NHS need?

Practice development that addresses the health needs of the local population

Practice should be appropriate for the needs of both individual patients and the wider population. For example, a practice nurse may be interested in the management of asthma, but if there are already enough nurses in the team with this kind of expertise then they would make a greater impact by concentrating on an aspect of unmet need – this might be the management of TB, care of the homeless or coronary heart disease management. Community nurses, midwives and health visitors are well placed to tackle inequalities in health. They will increasingly be asked to prioritise their work, develop their practice and target their efforts towards those in greatest need.

Practice development that turns strategy into action

Health improvement programmes are the vehicles for developing strategies that will improve health and reduce inequalities in health. They specify the range and location of, and investment in, health services and acknowledge the importance of partnership working with other statutory organisations and the voluntary sector. As such they are a valuable source of information for health professionals. Increasingly, care pathways will be designed to ensure that services are properly organised across the community, primary and secondary care sectors. National Service Frameworks also play a major role in the development of local services.

National and local strategies will increasingly challenge aspects of existing practice and generate great scope for new roles and different ways of delivering care. Practice development must support strategic goals. For example, midwives might be required to provide a service focused on the needs of women who misuse drugs – to do this effectively they will need to develop new knowledge and skills.

Effective practice development

Evidence-based practice involves systematically appraising and using up-to-date research findings for the basis of clinical decisions. Although there is a growing body of nursing and therapy research it is clear that, as for medicine, implementation of best practice is still patchy. Increased attention is being given to the development aspect of research and development in order to ensure that research findings are implemented. Major improvements could be achieved if all nurses applied best practice relating to infection control, continence care, tissue viability, palliative care, patient dignity and the safety of people with serious mental illness.

Efficient practice development

In a publicly funded and cash limited service we all have a duty to ensure that every pound of taxpayers' money is used efficiently. Every pound used unnecessarily carries an opportunity cost in that inefficiency in one area deprives other patients of care. Practice development should therefore demonstrate best value and help the NHS respond to the pressures that it is experiencing. This requirement challenges us to consider what level of quality is affordable and desirable in different clinical arenas. Naturally we all aspire to the gold standard but if the financial cost of this deprives another service of the resources needed to maintain a safe service then it is necessary to settle for the optimum standard. For example, some would like to see waiting lists for surgical treatment reduced to a maximum of six months. However, implementation of this standard across the board would be so expensive that there would be little or no money available to fund other aspects of health care such as mental health or community services. Choices must be made based on a judgement about the best use of available funding.

Efficient practice and practice development usually require teamwork and a willingness to do things differently. Clinical staff are best placed to work out the most cost effective way to achieve satisfactory outcomes. Many service improvements depend upon shifts in practice across traditional professional and organisational boundaries, for example 'Hospital at Home Schemes' demonstrate the scope for caring for people in their own home rather than hospital in certain circumstances. An initiative of this kind requires close collaboration between the patient and their informal carers, nurses, hospital clinicians, GPs, therapists and managers. NHS staff must also work in partnership with Local Authority caring support teams. In future there will be more multi-professional learning and teaching to support patient-centred practice.

Practice development that maintains safety

Many people feel extremely vulnerable when they access health care. They place their trust in NHS professionals and have a right to expect that everyone involved in their care will be competent. Health professionals have a duty to keep up-to-date and maintain quality standards. Public confidence can quickly be eroded.

High quality may have a high cost but so does poor quality. In financial terms this is, for example, associated with delayed recovery and hence extended length of stay either in hospital or on a community nursing caseload; unnecessary readmission; the time dedicated to investigating complaints and the enormous costs of litigation. In non-financial terms the costs may also be immense, for example the pain associated with a pressure sore or hospital acquired infection, disability following a fracture obtained as a result of an avoidable fall, disease caused by major drug errors, injury to the mentally ill patient or the public where risk assessment procedures have failed. In extreme cases quality failures can lead to avoidable death. National Audit reports along with a number of high profile cases have exposed major flaws in both clinical practice and management within the NHS. These seriously erode public confidence and increase our responsibility to put in place systems that support safe practice and reduce the scope for mistakes happening.

In addition to creating a framework for improving and maintaining performance, clinical governance also requires the NHS to identify and deal with poor performance. There is a bottom line below which care must be considered unacceptable. Managers will need to support practice development at both the leading edge and the trailing edge – hopefully moving every aspect of practice forward over time and narrowing the gap between the best and the worst.

Health professionals must audit and critically appraise their own practice and that of their colleagues. The goal should be to identify and resolve potential problems early on – before standards slip to a dangerous level. Support should be offered to help raise standards – this is an important aspect of practice development. The ability to 'learn through doing' and to overcome weaknesses in a supportive environment is part of a learning culture.

How will clinical governance support practice development?

The introduction of clinical governance could be viewed as the most radical part of the latest reforms or, indeed, any of the reforms since the birth of the NHS. This is the first time that Chief Executives have had a statutory responsibility for quality. It is also the first time that professional self-regulation has been seriously challenged and asked to demonstrate its ability to systematically deliver safe care and maintain public confidence.

Practice development right across the performance curve is one of the core aspects of clinical governance. Nurses and other health professionals have been firm supporters of structured practice development programmes and these are well-established in some organisations. However, corporate support for implementing structures and systems that support this initiative has not always been forthcoming. It is extremely difficult for even the most determined and innovative practitioner to make progress in the absence of leadership from the top of the organisation. Passion alone cannot implement and sustain radical change, structures and systems are needed too. Clinical governance will support practice development within every NHS organisation. This is however a major change programme which will take time to become fully established. Organisations must regularly evaluate their current performance and produce organisational development action plans. These will focus on the structures and systems required to secure effective governance. Consideration must also be given to creating a culture within which clinical governance will flourish. Some of the key considerations are summarised below.

Organisational structures and systems

Having been given statutory responsibility for quality of care chief executives must be confident that the organisation will:

* identify and build on good practice
* identify, assess and minimise the risk of untoward incidents
* ensure that lessons are learned when things go wrong and deal with poor clinical performance
* support health professionals in delivering quality care.

Effective clinical governance will depend on synthesising many different strands of existing work along with the introduction of some new tasks. Research and development, clinical audit, clinical effectiveness, complaints management, risk management, patient information, continuing professional education and training, performance review, clinical leadership, supervision and resource management are all important. Bench-marking enables managers and clinicians to compare standards across different organisations and share achievements. Because the agenda is large and time is limited, it will be important for staff to identify priorities for action. It may, for example, be helpful to consider the following questions:

* Which aspects of practice development would have the greatest impact on the quality of care for the population served? (Be relentless in pursuing high standards in basic aspects of care such as infection control.)
* What are the main areas of clinical risk in the team or organisation?
* Which services will be changed for other reasons in the near

future? (Practice development should be built-in to change management rather than bolted-on at a later stage and it is usually easier to change something where the status quo has been unfrozen.)

- Which aspects of practice already have a sound evidence base? (Implementation of this may be more worthwhile than embarking on totally new ventures.)
- Who will be ambassadors for specific aspects of practice development? (Identify, develop and harness their skills and influence then celebrate and publicise success.)
- What aspects of good practice already exist in the organisation? Have these been properly implemented in all other areas? If not, why not?

Information from every part of the organisation is needed to produce the Trust's monthly and annual quality report. Good information systems are very important in that they enable staff to capture accurate, timely and relevant data.

Quality improvement processes will clearly have an important role to play. Clinical staff are already required to participate in clinical audit and in future this should become a mainstream activity. Results will routinely be presented to the Trust Board enabling satisfactory performance to be acknowledged; where problems are identified chief executives will expect further exploration of the casual factors so that action can be taken to close the loop. Peer review, external audit and clinical supervision are other examples of quality improvement processes. Practice development will often be one of the interventions used to improve standards of care.

Continuing professional development (CPD) is central to high quality patient care. All registered nurses, midwives and health visitors have to undertake continuing professional development to be able to renew their registration every three years. National guidance (DoH, 1998a and 1999d) extends this requirement to all clinicians, sets out expectations of the NHS and the timetable for implementation. CPD is already well-established in many organisations but now **all** health organisations must implement local arrangements to ensure that robust arrangements are in place. In future every health professional will agree with their manager a plan that will enable them to keep up-to-date and develop their practice. Plans must meet local service needs as well as the aspirations of individuals. Work-based learning will have a valuable role to play as will distance learning and more formal programmes of professional education and training.

Continuing professional development should build on previous knowledge, experience and skills, and enhance the ability to interpret and apply knowledge based on research and development. It lies at the heart of professionalism and involves much more than going on a course. The CPD framework will support professionals in their desire to constantly enhance practice. The new structured approach required of employers will ensure that **all** staff participate in lifelong learning.

Organisational cultures

The concept of culture is difficult to define. Hampden-Turner (1990) describes culture as,

... a whole way of life, ways of acting, feeling and thinking, which are learned by groups of people rather than being biologically determined.

Deal and Kennedy (1988) simply define culture as,

The way we do things round here.

When collaboration is desired between different groups or organisations the likely interplay between the different cultures must be considered and managed (Carnal, 1990). A number of authors, including Peters and Waterman (1982), Hofstede (1991) and Ourousoff (1992) have noted the importance of organisational culture. Although the debate about the extent to which corporate culture can be changed is still underway there is general agreement that it has a profound effect on both efficiency and morale. It influences the way in which strategic decisions are made, how change is managed and also how routine work is undertaken.

Clinical governance is likely to flourish in organisations that:

+ are patient and service focused
+ value and promote partnership working and collaboration
+ engage staff in change management and actively promote professional development and life-long learning
+ establish clear accountability arrangements
+ set explicit and achievable standards, monitor performance and introduce transparent reporting systems
+ empower individuals and teams to overcome obstacles to change
+ foster leadership at all levels
+ celebrate success
+ address poor performance consistently and fairly.

Although it is essential to ensure that poor standards of care are properly addressed, clinical governance is not about searching for bad apples. It is about creating a learning culture that nurtures reflective practice and recognises the importance of learning through doing. This clearly requires effective clinical leadership.

The richer picture

The introduction of clinical governance is a very logical and long overdue initiative. It will provide a framework in which practice development can flourish. It represents a challenge to every organisation. The fabric of the NHS is woven from a rich mixture of professional cultures and traditions. Power and influence do not always work in the way organisational charts suggest. There are therefore a number of issues and questions that deserve further consideration.

Managing the tension between clinical freedom and corporate accountability

Self-regulation is a privilege enjoyed by professional groups who must now demonstrate their ability to place the safety of patients above the needs of their members. Although chief executives have a statutory duty for quality, professional bodies wield a considerable amount of power. How will chief executives fulfil their obligations for clinical governance in organisations where clinicians resist external monitoring? Will professional bodies support managers who require non-participating clinicians to fall into line? How should practice be evaluated and by whom?

Achieving the right balance between support and collusion

It is essential to create a culture that enables people to declare and learn from their mistakes. A blame culture will lead to resistance to change. However there is a risk that this rationale could be used to avoid taking firm action when seriously poor performance has been identified. A seemingly facilitative culture can easily become a complacent and collusive culture. How can organisations achieve the right balance?

Securing the resources

Although there are undoubtedly financial savings to be made through the eradication of poor practice it is unlikely that these will fund the cost of evening out practice to the desired standard right across the country. In practice, the implementation of clinically effective care is likely to require additional money. The extra resources needed to improve quality of the existing level of provision will obviously compete with the demand for new and faster services along with new drugs and technology

It is the duty of professionals to use NHS resources wisely, however politicians also have a duty to shape public expectations, establish relative priorities and make the necessary level of funding available. Prioritisation is a sensitive political issue as is taxation. Will politicians have the courage to enter into this debate and will the public be prepared to pay higher taxes should this be necessary?

Involving the public in a meaningful way

Everyone accepts that it is important to engage the public in the development of health strategies, to seek their views on local services and to share information about the NHS in an open way. At national level the public are represented on both the National Institute of Clinical Excellence and the Commission for Health Improvement.

The views of patients and carers and the wider population are often sought by Health Authorities and NHS Trusts when services are being reviewed. Community Health Councils are often represented on corporate quality groups; many wards and departments have introduced innovative ways of getting feedback on services provided. It is less clear what information should be shared with the public about local standards of care and the best way of communicating this.

How open should we be? Should we develop and publish league tables in the local press, eg. of pressure sore, infection and re-admission rates? What about details of serious incidents and near misses? At what level of aggregation should data be shared with the public? Individual clinician, team, or across the whole organisation? Who should have access to clinical audit results? How might we help the public to interpret bench-marking data? How can we hope to engage anxious staff in clinical audit in a non-threatening way if we simultaneously expose them to (possibly harsh and unfair) public scrutiny and media criticism? What effect would this have on public confidence? What impact would it have on staff morale? These questions illustrate the importance of adopting a considered and sensitive approach to this important issue.

Governance across boundaries

Care will increasingly be provided by multi-professional and multi-agency teams whose members will be accountable to different organisations operating different quality assurance systems, for example, in community mental health teams. How will clinical governance work in these circumstances? The concept of 'virtual organisations' is an interesting one and the removal of artificial demarcations will be essential if we are to deliver patient-centred care. However, 'virtual' accountability is unacceptable and care must be taken to remove ambiguity when new partnership ventures are established.

What next?

Full implementation of clinical governance must be seen as a massive change management programme. It will take years to achieve, and as illustrated above, there are a number of issues that will need further attention. It offers a great opportunity to improve standards of care, boost public confidence and professional morale. It is important to recognise that practice development does not, and should not, exist in isolation. It is a central plank of health care strategy and clinical governance. Quality is everyone's business — whatever their role or grade. Everyone can make a contribution to improving standards of care, most importantly at the level of personal practice and also more widely within their organisation. Some aspects of change management require considerable effort and organisational support, others can quite easily be achieved by an individual who feels motivated to develop their practice and is prepared to take a few personal risks. Consider the following suggestions:

1. Contribute to setting, and understand the goals of your team. Ask some challenging questions. What are the health needs of the people you serve? How equitable is the service? How effective is it? Are there aspects of practice that should be stopped? How efficient is it? Where are the

gaps? What are the main areas of clinical and non-clinical risk? How strong is the team? What is staff morale like? How are all of these things measured?

2. Ask a patient and/or their carer to tell you about the best and worst aspects of the care that you have given them in the last week – thank them for their help, reflect upon their responses and form a plan to build on the best and sort out the rest. Make this a routine part of your practice.

3. Ask your manager, your clinical supervisor, a senior doctor with whom you work, three members of your peer group and three junior team members to give you candid feedback on your performance, ask, for example: What are my strengths? What are my weaknesses? What helpful personal qualities do I bring to the team? How might I make a stronger contribution? Recognise that this feedback is very subjective but reflect on it and use it to accelerate your personal and professional development, talk it over with your clinical supervisor, make notes of key learning points in a reflective diary and build practical actions into your personal development plan (this kind of feedback is contagious, soon everyone will be doing it).

4. Ask a respected colleague to 'shadow' you and observe what you do either for half an hour or for an hour while you undertake a specific procedure or for a shift – whatever is manageable – ask for specific observations and comments. Be prepared to offer them the same support.

5. Get into the habit of giving and receiving feedback.

6. Read a book on change management – your library will have many to choose from.

7. Ask your manager if you can 'shadow' them for a shift sometime over the next month so that you can gain insight into their role.

8. Ask your manager if you can arrange to spend a couple of days with a different team in your organisation (or even in a different organisation) – compare their practice with that of your team, return with at least three good ideas – build up your professional network.

9. Read the policy documents relating to your team. Are they all up-to-date, relevant, and helpful? How are they updated in your organisation?

10. Review record keeping in your area – either your own, or that of the team. Does it match up to the standard? What is the standard?

11. Participate in, or lead an aspect of clinical audit – get support from the specialist 'best practice' team within your organisation (if there isn't one, suggest this development to your manager).

12. Identify an aspect of practice that really interests you – preferably one that affects a large proportion of your patients – and aim to become more expert in it.

13. Ensure that you have a personal development plan and regular appraisal – this should drive practice development.

14. Become more directly involved in implementing clinical governance, for example, by reviewing progress within your team and the wider organisation. Ask your director of nursing for a copy of the baseline assessment checklist used for the organisation and apply this tool in your area of practice.

15. Help to formulate a development plan based on this assessment – make the connections between the different elements. Identify practical things that can be easily achieved in the early stages, concentrate on the basics, seek support, involve the multi-professional team.

16. Clarify accountability arrangements within your team.

17. Find out what the local Health Improvement Programme says about your service and check that you are implementing action required. Offer to contribute, even in a small way, to the production of the next version.

18. Attend a board meeting – consider what greater contribution you could make to your organisation.

19. Imagine what you would do differently if you were the chief executive of your organisation and how you would set about this – consider how you might use your influence more effectively within the organisation.

20. Identify one or more role models – and act as one.

21. Ensure that your IT skills are up-to-date and that you understand the need for the collection of data and contribute to the local evaluation of it.

Conclusion

This chapter has summarised some of the key developments in national policy in order to illustrate the links between clinical governance and practice development. Quality has always been at the heart of clinical practice. Most clinicians understand their accountability for maintaining and improving standards of care, however, for the first time in the history of the NHS, quality is now firmly on the agenda of every NHS organisation.

Clinical governance arrangements have been introduced to help rebuild confidence in the NHS as a public service, accountable to patients, open to the public and shaped by their views. In this climate organisations will recognise the importance of practice development that meets the needs of the target population, turns strategy into action and promotes safe, effective and efficient practice. Action must be taken to create structures and systems that will orchestrate many different stands of development work within an organisational culture that actively promotes the consistent achievement of sensitive, efficient and clinically effective care.

It will take some time for clinical governance to become fully established and in doing so further consideration must be given to a number of complex issues. These include reconciling the tension between clinical freedom and corporate accountability, managing the resource implications for the NHS, achieving the right balance between support and collusion, involving the public in a meaningful way and maintaining crisp accountability within complex teams.

The new quality agenda offers great opportunities for clinical staff to develop their practice. It is however important to recognise that the reforms may make some people feel threatened and vulnerable. Confident clinicians are highly skilled at helping patients to cope with major life changes; they now have an opportunity to support colleagues through change.

It is usually helpful for us to understand the larger picture and then identify what our personal contribution can be. There are many practical things that can be done by individuals who choose to exercise leadership within their sphere of practice.

10

Power, influence and control in practice development

Dr Richard Byrt

Who has the power, influence and control in practice development? The answer is complex for several reasons. Firstly, it depends on how power, influence and control are defined. Secondly, the literature suggests that a wide variety of factors influence the development of practice. There are relevant findings from studies in health service and social policy, management, organisational theory, sociology, psychology, law and the history and development of health service professions and professional-client relationships. Also relevant are feminist, gay and lesbian studies and research on ethnicity and disablement (Wilkinson and Miers, 1999a).

After a brief overview, this chapter will consider the meaning of power, influence and control and related concepts of empowerment and participation. It will then examine practice development in relation to individual service users and practitioners, the health service organisation and wider social and political factors. The chapter will conclude by considering these areas in relation to the nursing care of people whose mental health problems are associated with seriously aggressive or offending behaviours.

As a form of convenient shorthand, the terms service user and practitioner will be used. The latter term usually refers to nurses and/or midwives, unless otherwise specified.

Factors influencing practice development

There is evidence that individuals both influence and are influenced by the social groups and societies of which they are a part (Robinson, 1993). *Figure 10.1* illustrates the many factors in wider society and in health service organisations which influence practice development, and which service users and practitioners may themselves influence to bring about change. Practice development in the present is affected, in part, by historical factors and by the goals and aspirations of the individuals involved. 'There are social, economic and political factors that run through historical periods and form direct links between the past and present' (Godsell, 1999).

Figure 10.1: Factors influencing practice development: individual, organisational and wider society

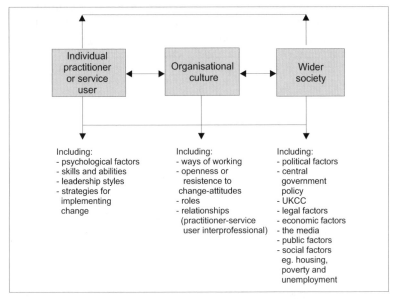

Before considering the influence of these individual, organisational and wider social factors on practice development, the nature of power, influence and control will be examined.

Power

Power is a complex concept, which has many meanings, depending on the perspective of the sociologist or political theorist (Philp, 1996; Masterson and Maslin-Prothero, 1999; Wilkinson, 1999). According to Philp (1996), 'power is concerned with the bringing about of consequences'. It is important to note that social scientists disagree about more rigorous definitions of the concept. Masterson and Maslin-Prothero (1999) comment,

> *... power in the political sense is usually taken to mean the ability to make other people do what you want them to do... Within the policy arena, power refers to the process by which*

the values and interests of one group are acted upon over and above the values and interests of another...

Philp (1996) refers to different bases of power, eg. an individual's 'status, knowledge, charisma', ways in which power is used to achieve particular ends and 'different forms of power', eg. influence, coercion and control. Wilkinson and Miers (1999b) give an overview of critiques of professional power by various sociologists, including those with feminist, Marxist and functionalist perspectives.

Influence

Handy (1993) states that within work organisations,

... influence is the process whereby A seeks to modify the attitudes and behaviour of B. Power is that which enables him to do it.

Handy refers to various methods of influence. Among the most relevant to practice development are rules and procedures, persuasion and magnetism, which originate from the individual's expertise or personality. A service user or junior practitioner might have little power, in relation to her/his role in the organisation, but be able to considerably influence practice development because of knowledge, commitment or enthusiasm. Other types of influence include the use of force, exchange (including the ability to bargain from ownership of resources) and 'manipulating the physical and psychological environment to achieve certain purposes' (Handy, 1993 as cited by Senior, 1997). Senior (1997) comments that, in work organisations, power and influence overlap, and are not as easy to distinguish as Handy suggests.

Handy's description of influence reflects, in part, the concept of social influence in social psychology.

A social influence process involves behaviour by one person that has the effect – or ... the intention – of changing the way another person behaves, feels or thinks about a stimulus.

Zimbardo and Leippe, 1991

Of relevance to practice development are studies of leadership styles and how and why people conform (Smith, 1995; Zimbardo and Leippe, 1991).

Control

The concept of control can be applied to practice development in two ways. In the sense used by social psychologists (Försterling, 1995), control can refer to the actual extent that service users and practitioners are able to cause particular changes in practice to happen. It can also be used to describe their beliefs that they are able to cause such changes (Tones, 1998).

In addition, social control is a concept used by sociologists to refer to 'practices developed by social groups of all kinds which enforce or encourage conformity and deal with behaviour which violates accepted norms' (Jary and Jary, 1995). The concept of social control has relevance to practice development because people in health service organisations may exert strong pressure on individuals who are developing practice to behave in particular ways. However, Dingwall *et al* (1988) point out that social control is not necessarily oppressive and may enable individuals to work together.

Examples of power, influence and control in practice development will be considered later in this chapter.

Empowerment and participation

The extent to which individual service users and practitioners can contribute to practice development depends, in part, on the extent to which they are empowered and enabled to participate (Kendall, 1998a; Øvretveit, 1997; Wilkinson and Miers, 1999b). Most authors' definitions of empowerment include reference to the transfer of power from one 'individual or group to another'(Gibson, 1995) and/or enabling individuals to take action or develop control over factors which affect them (Fraher and Limpinnian, 1999; Kendall, 1998b; Ryles, 1999).

Empowerment is often reflected in participation: the involvement of individuals or groups (usually recipients of a service) in decision-making and responsibility in areas which affect their own lives. Examples of participation include the involvement of service users and grassroots staff in decisions concerning individual care or health service policy (Byrt, 1994; McFadyen and Farrington, 1997; Tones, 1998).

Both empowerment and participation are complex, multi-faceted phenomena which exist at different **degrees** and **levels**. **Degrees** refer to the amount of participation or exercise of power, which (as illustrated in *Figure 10.2*) may range from being given information to the total running of an organisation. Levels of participation vary from decisions made by a service user and/or practitioner about aspects of individual care, to involvement in decision-making at the Department of Health (Byrt, 1994; McFadyen and Farrington, 1997).

Figure 10.2: Degrees and levels of participation and empowerment

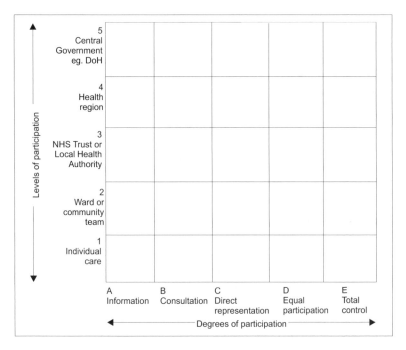

It is suggested that the relationship between power and participation in practice development is circular (*Figure 10.3*). The degree and level of participation of service users and practitioners is dependant, in part, on the extent to which they are perceived by others and by themselves to have power, influence and control. In addition, active participation in practice development may (sometimes, but not invariably) increase participants' personal experience of empowerment and the extent to which they are seen as having specific power, eg. the expertise and knowledge to make changes.

Figure 10.3: Relationship between participation and empowerment

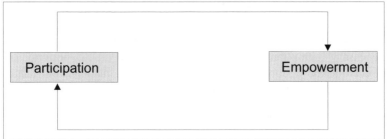

The relationship of individual, organisational and social factors in practice development

The literature suggests that individual, organisational and wider social factors all contribute to practice development and that their effects are interconnected. *The Health of the Nation* (DoH, 1992a) emphasised the importance of individuals taking personal responsibility for their health, but, unlike the more recent *Our Healthier Nation* (DoH, 1998b, cited in Fatchett, 1998), made little reference to the effect on health of wider social factors such as poverty, poor housing and unemployment. Tones (1998) comments that,

> ... [a] *culture of poverty will limit capacity for healthy action... Empowered individuals will have a greater chance of changing their circumstances, but those same circumstances will limit their opportunity for self-empowerment.*

The power, influence and control of the individual in practice development

Research suggests that one factor involved in successful practice development is clarity about who should be involved as participants, and the degree and level of their participation (Byrt, 1994; McFadyen and Farrington, 1997). In certain circumstances, it may be more effective to gradually increase the participation in practice development of service users and junior staff in incremental stages, beginning with the giving of information and consultation, and increasing participation at higher levels once participants' confidence has increased.

In addition, experience of participation in practice development at an individual level would probably be necessary in order to develop confidence to participate at higher levels, eg. Trust board, Health Authority or Department of Health. This would be particularly necessary with clients or junior nurses who had little experience of, or confidence in, contributing to decisions about the delivery of care. An example would be a group of older people or individuals with learning disabilities with (sadly) limited experience of choice or non-institutionalised environments (Byrt, 1994).

Some service users and practitioners may feel powerless to influence practice development at Trust board or higher levels. If this is the case, it may be possible for them to develop practice at the level of individual care, even within limited resources. One example is recent work which seeks to counter people's lack of acknow-ledgement of the identities and roles of older individuals with Alzheimer's disease, and the failure to attempt to understand the value and meanings of their communications (Bender and Cheston, 1997; Downe, 1997; Small et al, 1998). Cameron (1998) gives a moving account of her efforts, as a health care support worker, to increase her understanding of the perspectives and experiences of these people and to develop practice in this area.

A number of psychological factors have been found to be associated with an individual's effective action to improve their own health. These include feelings of self-empowerment, with con-comitant high levels of self-esteem and self-efficacy. The latter refers to an individual's judgement that she/he is capable of bringing about a desired outcome, eg. maintaining regular exercise in order to lose weight (Tones, 1998; Tones and Tilford, 1994). Latter (1998) found that medical ward nurses with the highest amounts of 'personal efficacy, competence, self-sufficiency and self-esteem' were more empowered and better able to make changes in nursing practice over which they experienced autonomy and control.

There is evidence that the individual's ability to influence others, and to provide leadership and management, is crucial in effecting change. The appropriate type of leadership depends on the type of organisation, its aims and culture (Handy, 1993) and the particular change strategy being implemented. Choice of the latter relates to what is to be changed, the reasons for the change, and its planning, implementation and evaluation (Wright, 1998a). For example, in order to make urgent changes in a ward with unsatisfactory nursing practice, a new Ward Manager might initially need a directive or *'telling'* (Keyzer and Wright, 1998) style of leadership, making clear decisions about standards of care, and ensuring through the power (legitimate authority), invested in her/his role, that these were met. However, a democratic or *'participating'* (Keyzer with Wright, 1998) style of leadership might be more effective in ensuring continuous development and improvements in practice, which are owned by both patients and staff.

There is debate among nursing historians about the extent to which past practice developments have been inspired by charismatic leaders, such as Florence Nightingale, rather than influenced by lesser-known nurses and other people (Rafferty, 1996). Issues such as class and ethnicity may affect which people are seen as having the power and influence to develop practice (Marks, 1997). It has been argued, for example, that the contribution of Mary Seacole, a contemporary of Nightingale, has been little acknowledged because she was black (Johnson, 1999). Until recently, historical accounts have stressed the contributions of middle class women in London teaching hospitals, rather than those of working class men and women in workhouse infirmaries and asylums (Dingwall *et al*, 1988; Nolan, 1995).

There is some evidence that certain service users and practitioners have particularly influenced recent practice developments. These include pioneers of nursing development units, who appear to have made extensive contributions to the development of the *New Nursing* (Salvage and Wright, 1995; Wright, 1998b). In addition, many health service users and their carers have used their experiences and expertise to found voluntary organisations which have campaigned for health service improvements. These include the National Schizophrenia Fellowship, formed in 1972, primarily to provide support for informal carers of people with schizophrenia (Pringle, 1980); and the Matthew Trust, which campaigns for improvements in maximum security hospitals. The latter organisation was founded by Peter Thompson following his horrendous experiences as a patient at Broadmoor (Thompson, 1972).

While the work of many charismatic leaders has endured, some organisations, such as therapeutic communities, have dissolved, once their leaders have left. To ensure continued and effective practice development, charismatic (and other) leaders need to ensure that they have successors who can continue to further develop and improve practice (Manning, 1989).

Organisational factors in practice development

The health service, of which the individual service user or practitioner is a part, will also affect her/his efforts to develop practice. It is suggested that the term organisational culture can be used to include the roles and relationships of service users and staff, and the attitudes they have towards each other. According to Handy (1993) organisational culture is also:

> ... *a pervasive way of life, or set of norms, ... deep-set beliefs about the way work should be organised, the way authority should be exercised, people rewarded, people controlled... The customs and traditions of a place are a powerful way of influencing behaviour...*

There is evidence that practice development is influenced by the ways in which patients, nurses and doctors are socialised (Wicks, 1998). While there was variation between different institutions, nurses in most settings tended, from at least the mid-nineteenth century until recently, to be socialised into strict hierarchies, with clear rules and routines, where the orders of sister, matron and doctor were to be carried out without question. Such organisational environments may have been originally adopted as a response to indiscipline among some nurses before nineteenth century reforms, and to ensure high standards of nursing care at a time when fewer treatments were available (Baly, 1995).

Unquestioning obedience to superiors' orders may have had advantages at a time when good nursing, in the absence of any alternatives, was essential to save life or prevent some people with mental illness or learning disabilities from seriously harming themselves or others (Baly, 1995; Nolan, 1995). However, a possible legacy was the development, well into the second half of the twentieth century, of routinised and ritualised nursing practices, 'because Sister says so', instead of practice development, based on reflection and research findings and in collaboration with service users (Walsh and Ford, 1989). Some settings, particularly those caring for older people, or individuals with mental health problems or learning disabilities, become institutionalised, with routines to ensure completion of tasks. This displaced the meeting of clients' individual needs and enabling their active participation in care (Barton, 1959; Morris, 1969; Robb, 1967).

In addition, practice and its development, like wider society, has often failed to take into account the needs and perspectives of people from ethnic minorities, women, lesbians and gay men and individuals with stigmatised diagnoses and disablements (Wilkinson and Miers, 1999). Examples include assumptions by mental health professionals that cultural beliefs are delusional (Littlewood and Lipsedge, 1997), nurses' prejudiced attitudes towards people with learning disabilities (Slevin and Sines, 1996) or who are living with AIDS (VÄLimÄKi *et al*, 1998), and failure to appreciate the needs of lesbians and gays and their partners (Godfrey, 1999).

The organisational cultures described above have not been conducive to practice development, and staff who have tried to protest or make changes have sometimes been ostracised or abused by colleagues (Martin, 1984; Pilgrim, 1995; Wright, 1998a). In contrast, Wright (1998a) comments on present day requirements that Health Services change, adding,

...changing practice at clinical level has difficulty in expanding or progressing if the total organisation has not accepted the culture of change. It does not render change impossible, but it does produce limitations. The change agent must be aware of these factors in order to limit the obstructions they can present, limit the damage that can be done, and how to overcome or get around them.

Some health service organisations have been set up with the intention of creating cultures where change can readily occur. These include nursing development units, which are centres 'for creative nursing, where change is planned and accepted as a way of life, where nursing practices are soundly based, but open constantly to change and review' (Wright, 1998b). Therapeutic communities aim to create 'cultures of enquiry' (Hinshelwood, 1999). These enable residents to learn about themselves and their relationship difficulties, express and resolve painful feelings and problems, and discover and develop positive attributes and abilities (Byrt, 1999). Both therapeutic communities and nursing development units stress the importance of resident/patient active participation in care and the provision of support, supervision and education for staff (Campling and Davies, 1997; Wright, 1998b).

The extent to which lecturers, researchers and quality co-ordinators in nursing and midwifery can influence practice development, depends on the relevance of their activities to practice. Much has been written about 'theory-practice' and 'research-practice' gaps (Rolfe, 1998c). More recently, there have been moves away from separation to an integration of nursing practice, research, education and quality (*Figure 10.4*), with the appointment of joint clinical/ university posts and increases in lecturers' time in clinical areas (Stitt, 1995). Nursing development units, in particular, endeavour to apply research and audit findings to practice and vice versa, often through action research (Salvage and Wright, 1995; Wright, 1998b). The appointment of appropriate staff and development of effective procedures and committees and procedures for Audit, in order to develop practice, has been stressed (Miles et al, 1996).

Figure 10.4: Separation and integration of nursing practice and nursing research, quality and education

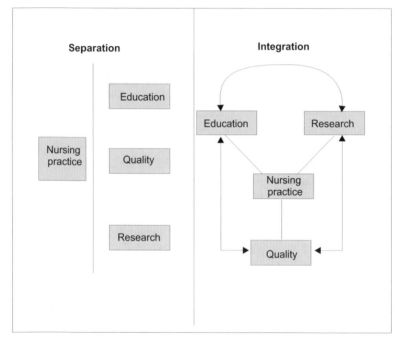

Despite some variations, research findings indicate that, in general, doctors have had greater power in decision-making in practice development compared with nurses, midwives and service users. It has been argued that this is partly because of the dominance of a predominantly male profession over ones which are mainly female, and whose knowledge base has less status (Shirley and Mander, 1996; Wicks, 1998). Recent increases in the proportion of female medical students and developments in professionalisation and education among midwives and nurses may change this (Wicks,

1998). In addition, there has been a number of successful challenges by service users, nurses and midwives to medical hegemony. An example is given later in this chapter.

Wider social factors and their influence on practice development

NHS Trusts, District Health Authorities, Health Regions and the Department of Health have a certain amount of power and control to develop practice. In addition, while most power, influence and control exerted by service users and practitioners are at the lower levels of participation (see *Figure10.2*), they have often exerted influence (sometimes successfully) at higher levels, particularly on some Trust Boards and the Department of Health.

Under Conservative administrations from 1979, Central Government's influence on practice at lower levels of the organisation was sometimes limited. For example, in the mid- nineteen seventies, money was allocated by the then Department of Health and Social Security to Regional Health Authorities to establish medium secure units. Several regions spent this money on other services instead (Gostin, 1985). From 1979 the Department of Health has made more active efforts to influence practice and in some cases has used legislation to compel managers of local services to make (sometimes considerable) changes (Fatchett, 1998).

Under Conservative Governments, the introduction of General Management in 1983, and NHS Trusts in 1989, met with considerable opposition from nurses and other professionals. The reforms considerably weakened the power of nurses and resulted in a marked reduction in the number of nurse managers. However, by the late eighties, 'nursing staff had gained some representation in the general management hierarchy' (Fatchett, 1998). During the eighties and early nineties, many nursing posts were lost or downgraded with considerable cuts in services. The latter included the closure of the Oxford Nursing Development Unit. This was without explanation, despite research evidence that its developments in practice had resulted in increased improvements in nursing care, greater patient satisfaction and independence, and lower treatment costs, compared with a control group (Pearson, 1995).

At this time, nurses' power and influence to develop practice appeared to be particularly affected by Department of Health policy,

... the expressed wish of the Government was to ensure that 'nurses' time was deployed to best effect on work which required special skills, leaving work which did not require these skills to be done by others'. This reflects... the early dissection and paring down of the professional role of the nurse by others who... fail to understand that nursing care is much more than providing technical skills and acting as assistants to doctors... the changes... reinforced a medicalised concept of health and health care, and this underpinned what the role of the nurse was to be within the reforming NHS. This in turn served to create... a fragmentation of care by nurses....

Fatchett, 1998

Whistleblowing

In the eighties and early nineties, many staff, including nurses, faced considerable difficulties when they drew managers' attention to resources and other problems which affected patient care. Their attempts to improve and develop practice through such whistle-blowing, including speaking out against changes and cuts in some Trusts, often resulted in dismissal and other penalties (Fatchett, 1998; Hunt, 1995).

Despite this, the UKCC made it clear that nurses, midwives and health visitors had accountability to report to senior managers any concerns about adverse effects of resource limitations on patient and client care (UKCC, 1989; UKCC, 1996b).

However, some Trusts have sought ways to inform and consult staff about changes, or have formulated strategies to increase the participation of service users and their informal carers (Central Nottinghamshire Healthcare NHS Trust, 1999; Leicestershire and Rutland NHS Trust, 1999). The White Paper *The new NHS modern – dependable* (DoH, 1997) stated the intention to make Trust board meetings open to the public and,

... to ensure... that Board membership is more representative of the local community...

DoH, 1997, quoted in Fatchett, 1998

Economic factors

In many cases, decisions affecting practice development appear to have been made primarily for economic reasons. Critics have argued that moves, from the mid-nineteen seventies, towards community-based, rather than institutional care, occurred largely to save money at a time of economic recession (Lewis and Glennerster, 1996). In the earlier days of NHS Trusts, an emphasis on economy was, in the view of some authors, at the expense of ensuring quality of services. *The new NHS modern – dependable* (DoH, 1997) while emphasising cost-effectiveness, shifted 'the focus onto quality of care, so that excellence is guaranteed to all patients' (DoH, 1997 quoted in Fatchett, 1998).

Some practitioners have seen the increased emphasis on cost-effectiveness in the NHS as an opportunity to develop practice, rather than a threat. While staff in therapeutic communities have experienced the reforms as antithetical to the principles by which they work (Campling and Davies, 1997), many have recently demonstrated the long term cost-effectiveness of therapeutic community treatment, and developed alternatives to expensive residential care, such as the application of therapeutic community principles to day services and provision in the community (Campling and Haigh, 1999).

Recent examples of Central Government's power over practice development include the setting up of the National Institute for Clinical Effectiveness, to ensure the development of clinically effective interventions, clinical governance, primary care groups and national surveys of the views of service users (DoH, 1997, cited in Fatchett, 1998; DoH, 1998a).

Influence of service users and practitioners on central government

The Department of Health frequently meets with a wide range of trade unions, professional and voluntary organisations concerned with the development of practice, and consults with specific service user and informal carer groups about various aspects of health (Department of Health, 1996). Traditionally, doctors have had greater influence on Central Government than nurses and service user groups. This became less true during Conservative administrations between

1979–1997, when many doctors campaigned against the Government (Cameron, 1999).

A distinction has been made between insider and outsider groups who lobby Central Government. Core insider groups include those, such as the British Medical Association, and Royal College of Midwives and Nursing, who are asked for their views by the Department of Health, on a wide range of health topics (Kingdom, 1991; Mahoney, 1994 cited by Cameron, 1999).

Many major charities, concerned with health, and representing the views of services users and informal carers, lobby the Department of Health in order to influence policy. However, others, including those with views which are unacceptable to the Government, are outsiders, marginalised, with no influence on the 'policy making community' (Cameron, 1999). Byrt (1994) studied a small radical mental health voluntary organisation, which took a Marxist perspective and advocated the total overthrow of traditional mental health services. He found that members of this organisation were unable to influence Central Government policy, despite their campaigning. In contrast, MIND and the National Schizophrenia Fellowship had greater influence.

An example of the power of both service users and professionals, in influencing Central Government, is the lobbying by mothers and midwives for the development of midwifery services in response to women's needs, rather than facilities controlled by (mainly male) obstetricians. This led to the establishment of a House of Commons Select Committee and the production of *Changing Childbirth* (DoH, 1993 cited in Gordon, 1998). In line with this White Paper, woman-centred services, including midwife-managed units were set up. In addition, midwives successfully campaigned for the removal of shackles from women prisoners in labour (Thomson, 1996).

Legal and professional accountability

Finally, practitioners' power to develop practice is constrained (and in some cases, enhanced) by legal requirements of a variety of Acts of Parliament, for example the Mental Health Act, 1983 (Leiba, 1998) and the Children Act, 1989 (Dimond, 1996a) and by issues of legal and professional accountability. One example is midwives' facilitation of water births.

Research by Hall and Holloway (1998) found that mothers felt that labour in water enabled them to be in control of the birth. Midwives wishing to develop practice in this area have professional accountability under the Midwives' *Rules and Code of Practice* (UKCC, 1998). In addition, legal and managerial accountability affect practice development in the use of water births. Some senior managers have not allowed midwives to practise in this way because Trust Boards 'would have no defence if a medical catastrophe were to occur' (Dimond, 1996b). Dimond (1996b) reports the case of two midwives who were disciplined for delivering a baby in water when the mother decided not to leave the bath.

The power to resist control

This chapter will close with an examination of ways in which a specific area of practice is affected by individual organisational and social factors. The area discussed is the nursing care of people with mental health problems and related physically aggressive or offending behaviours. This has been an especially difficult area for practice development. Problems relate to frequent differences in perspective between patient/client and nurse, specific organisational cultures and the influence and power of many organisations in wider society (*Figure 10.5*). The latter is much greater than in most areas of health care (Mason and Mercer, 1998).

Many critics have referred to the power of both institutional and community services to control (and, in some cases, coerce) mental health patients and clients with histories of aggression or offending (Mason and Mercer, 1998). Some of the control rests with the Magistracy and the Judiciary, which make decisions about the hospital admission of patients from the courts; and the Home Office, which is concerned with decisions concerning the leave, transfer and discharge of many of these individuals. The Home Office sometimes decides that patients, particularly those admitted under the Mental Health Act with 'psychopathic disorder', cannot be discharged, even though these patients and the staff all agree that no further treatment would be beneficial (Gunn and Taylor, 1995). In addition, the care of patients is also influenced by the Department of Health, Health Region and Trust policies and practice. For example, the speed with which patients can be transferred to settings of lower security depends on the number of beds available.

Figure 10.5: Factors affecting practice development in the nursing care of patients with physically aggressive and offending behaviours

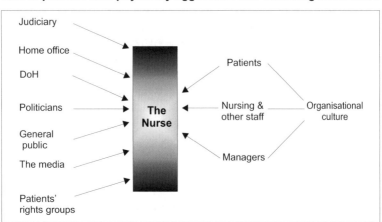

In addition, practice development in this area is particularly affected by public, political and media opinion. Some critics have commented that the Government's introduction of Supervision Orders, under the Mental Health (Care in the Community) Act, 1995, was a knee jerk response to considerable media and public pressure. This was in relation to a small number of incidents where mental health service users attacked or killed members of the public (McCann, 1998). Media images of people with mental health problems are usually negative, stigmatising and violent (Wahl, 1995), although the number of homicides committed by these individuals did not increase prior to the passing of the Mental Health (Care in the Community) Act, 1995 (Sayce, 1995).

Under this Act, the role of community mental health nurses in enforcing compliance with treatment, and (supposedly) ensuring public safety, has been seen as dis-empowering to clients and against their interests (Godin and Scanlon, 1997; McCann, 1998; Symonds, 1998, cited in Wells, 1998).

Organisational cultures

In addition, there have been extensive criticisms of maximum secure hospitals. Central Government enquiries at Rampton (DHSS, 1980) and The Ashworth Hospital (DoH, 1992b) found that practice development was hindered by their organisational cultures. At The

Ashworth, staff who attempted to challenge bad practice or introduce improvements, were treated as outsiders and threatened by colleagues. The Enquiry into this hospital found evidence of discriminatory attitudes towards patients and some staff. There was a close-knit, little changing, staff group. All these factors militated against effective practice development.

Various studies, as well as The Ashworth and Rampton Enquiries, have found that English maximum secure hospitals have been characterised by rules and preoccupations with security which have been unwarranted by patients' levels of dangerous behaviour (DHSS, 1980; DoH, 1992b; Mason and Mercer, 1998).

While earlier studies suggested that patients had relatively little power in mental health systems (Jones, 1993), more recent research has indicated ways in which they have been able to exert some power in their daily lives, even in secure settings. In his seminal work, *Asylums*, Goffman (1968) referred to patients' ability to 'work the system'. This included illicitly (from the staff's perspective) gaining extra material benefits and pretending to conform to staff expectations, in order to obtain discharge. Other authors have described clashes in patient and staff perspectives in maximum secure hospitals, with consequent adverse effects on practice development. Mercer (1998) refers to 'patients' rejection of an illness model and refusal to participate and co-operate' in these settings. Mason and Chandley (1990) described the difficulty of implementing nursing models in a maximum secure hospital, as patients did not see themselves as 'sick', and did not wish to engage in therapeutic relationships or collaborate with nurses in plans of care. Instead, many patients brought to the hospital a prison culture which worked in opposition to the goals of staff who were attempting to develop practice.

Developing practice

Despite all these difficulties, some authors have described ways of developing practice with this client/patient group. The present author's experience suggests that, in this, as in other areas, a first step in practice development is the identification of aspects of good practice, areas which need change or improvement, and priorities for development.

While negotiating common ground with clients/patients can be difficult, and should not be underestimated, research findings and accounts of nursing practice indicate that this is sometimes possible.

The problems of establishing engagement in treatment and a therapeutic alliance with people with severe anti-social and other personality disorders have been described. Understanding traumatic experiences of childhood abuse and neglect experienced by some of these individuals, and preparedness by staff to work with them and build up a trusting relationship, has been found to be beneficial (Campling, 1999; Norton and Hinshelwood, 1996).

Breeze and Repper (1998) found that clients with longstanding aggressive behaviours were more likely to engage in work with community mental health nurses, and were more satisfied if they could negotiate the care provided by the nurse.

Breeze and Repper (1998) distinguish between 'power over' clients, which the latter saw as unhelpful, and sharing 'power with' them: returning 'some control, to the patient and offer [ing] care and support which the patient recognises to be skilful and therapeutic'. Similarly, Lowe (1992) found that nurses considered that an important component of the care of patients with 'challenging behaviours' was enabling them not to lose face and to consider their feelings and perspectives.

Collins and Robinson (1997) examined how patients' privacy and dignity could be improved, within the parameters of safety, within a maximum secure hospital. Patients participated in the design of a questionnaire to investigate this. Effective solutions to the problem of maintaining both safety, and privacy and dignity of patients, were developed with them. Other secure hospital settings have also sought to effect improvements based on patients' views (McGregor-Kettles and Russell, 1997; Morrison *et al*, 1996). In the medium secure unit where the present author works, a patient satisfaction survey was planned in consultation with representatives from patients, the National Schizophrenia Fellowship, Leicestershire Community Health Council, the Unit's main purchaser and the Department of Nursing and Midwifery, De Montfort University. An action plan, based on areas of greatest patient dissatisfaction, was produced by Leicestershire Community Health Council. At the time of writing, this action plan is being implemented by managers and staff. Patients are being informed of progress, which will be monitored in other surveys. Such research can involve patients, as well as staff and managers, in the development of practice. However, it should be recognised that, despite such measures, the power of forensic patients is inevitably limited, as the majority has no choice but to be in secure provision.

Another crucial area of practice development concerns the care and management of patients/clients with physically aggressive behaviours. This includes preventing aggression and developing alternatives to seclusion, in an environment which encourages post-incident analysis and support, clinical supervision and education of staff (Alty, 1997; Mason and Chandley, 1999). Mason (1997) found that in one maximum security hospital, nurses tended to use seclusion, not to prevent physical harm to others, but because of concern about what managers and colleagues would think if they did not seclude.

Whittington and Balsamo (1998) have found, in research on aggressive incidents, that both power and fear, rather than being static,

... *flow from* [patient] *to the* [nurse] *and back, as the confrontation unfolds over minutes or even seconds.*

It is suggested by the present author that, in relation to physical aggression, both fear and lack of a sense of power, can prevent patients from establishing control over their behaviours; and nurses from providing effective care and management during such incidents. Learning effective strategies to cope with aggression may help nurses and patients to work together to develop practice in this area. For example, learning de-escalation techniques has been found to increase nurses' confidence (McHugh *et al*, 1995).

Various interventions have been found to help patients work with staff in order to express anger creatively, including those which use cognitive-behavioural and therapeutic community principles (Cullen *et al*, 1997; Tennant and Hughes, 1998).

The careful consideration of patients' perspectives and views, and the application of modified therapeutic community principles, may enable the questioning of aspects of organisational culture which inhibit practice development. Also of value, is working with voluntary organisations and local Community Health Councils, whose participants, as members of independent bodies, may observe areas for practice development which are not noticeable to staff who are closely involved in the organisation. A number of organisations have set up patients' councils and independent advocacy services in secure hospitals and units. WISH (Women in Secure Hospitals) met with considerable opposition from some managers and staff when it started its campaigns, in the mid-eighties, to improve services for women patients. It has recently become an accepted part of the 'policy making community' in the Department of Health and works actively with patients and staff to effect improvements in secure services for women (WISH, 1999).

Conclusion

This chapter has considered the many factors which affect practice development in relation to the individual service user or practitioner, health service organisational cultures and wider society, including Central Government policies. Examples of factors which facilitate or hinder practice development have been considered in relation to several areas of care. Both the present and the recent past have been examined.

Examples of practice development have also been considered. Often these have occurred despite, and sometimes in response to, many difficulties and challenges. In the words of Fatchett (1998), in relation to nursing:

> ... the many perceived and real barriers to professional development have singularly failed to halt the creation of innovative and relevant nursing responses to the ever-challenging health needs agenda. New skills have been developed in order to improve the standard of care offered... The future for professional nursing rests, not just within itself, but in a reciprocal partnership with the whole of the community.

Project-based practice development as a model

Ann Jackson

Introduction

Project-based practice development is a distinct approach currently being used within mental health. The development of this approach follows on from previous work undertaken with the RCN Institute (Ward, 1995; Kitson *et al*, 1996, Ward *et al,* 1998). Practice development work has been described as a process for establishing an evidence base through the development of new theoretical or experiential insights (Cutcliffe et al, 1998). Practice development might be said to be evident where these insights are articulated and are demonstrably contributing to a deliberate nursing practice. The extent to which 'evidence' should be, and can be, the basis for contemporary practice is, of course, under vigorous debate (Estabrooks, 1998). Clearly, the whole evidence-based movement is not without its difficulties, particularly in relation to questions about what counts as evidence? and whose evidence is taken as being legitimate? (Clarke, 1999).

More positively perhaps, this shift can provide the nurse/ practitioner with the opportunity to explore and consider a range of 'knowledge' and 'evidence' when making decisions about what might be deemed as 'best practice' or 'practice development'. Developing or establishing an evidence base to practice which is meaningful and relevant to both nurses and patients is an aspiration of all practice development supervised by the mental health project practice development team (MHPPDT). To say 'aspiration' is more honest and realistic as, in practice, this can be difficult to achieve.

In response to a demand for nurses to engage with, and implement, 'evidence-based' or 'best practice' initiatives, the MHPPDT have constructed a structured and supervised Programme of Practice Development. The most commonly undertaken programme is for a period of two years and formally provides an opportunity for a team of nurses to access and utilise relevant research findings and/or evidence; to employ appropriate research methods in the collection of local data/evidence; to lead and manage a practice change effectively; and to engage in activity which seeks to raise critical awareness and develop reflective practice. These activities are carried out over the two years within a defined project in order to maintain the focus on a specific area of practice and at the same time maximise the potential for the project to be sustained until the end. Agreeing future development after the formal 'end' then becomes another cycle of development for the project teams, their clinical areas and the organisation.

Underlying themes

Before describing the process for project-based practice development, it is necessary to briefly mention four main 'themes' which have informed the activities or processes that we consider fundamental to practice development, and have been described more fully elsewhere (Jackson *et al,* 1999a). The four themes are:

1. Our existing knowledge relating to the non-utilisation of research findings (Hunt, 1981; Luker, 1992; Closs and Cheater, 1994; Mulhall, 1995.) More recently, Parahoo (1999) has highlighted some pertinent issues in relation to research utilisation in psychiatric nursing.

2. The type of research methodologies and methods that are chosen by the programme participants to evaluate their practice and in some way describe or 'measure' their work. They are encouraged in the programme to consider the most appropriate methods for the questions that are important to them and their client group (Atkins, 1993).

3. Developing an awareness of the complexities of leading and managing 'bottom-up' change (Harvey, 1991). The successful practice developer faces a challenge in developing those skills, which engage their colleagues and can lead to effective and sustainable change within their clinical area (Waterman *et al,* 1995).

4. Raising critical awareness, developing critical thinking and reflexivity. Our understanding of this critical approach is informed by those principles shared with critical social research, action research and feminist methodologies. In order for project participants to 'become critical', facilitation is required to challenge

contradictions, assumptions and traditions in practice. Through reflection on individual and collective values (Nolan and Grant, 1993), roles and responsibilities can be clarified in response to new understandings (Carr and Kemmis, 1986).

Setting up projects

The MHPPDT currently supervises a wide range of projects (Jackson *et al* 1999b). Each project within a two-year programme of practice development is led by a 'project leader' and supported by two or more 'buddies'. Each project team comes from the clinical area where the practice issue has been agreed through a formal process of selection and where organisational funding and support has been established (Jackson *et al*, 1999a). *Figure 11.1* illustrates the range of 'key relationships' that we consider to be essential in setting up projects and need to be nurtured during the entire programme.

The criteria for projects that we consider to be viable can be seen in *Table 11.1*. These criteria help to put some manageable boundaries on the types of projects that are possible within the given time-frame of two years. It provides potential participants with a guide to some principles that, in our experience, are more likely to result in a sustainable project.

Figure 11.1: Key relationships in practice development

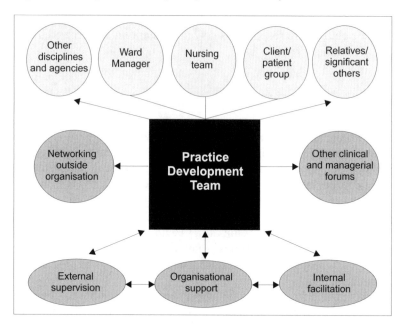

Table 11.1: Issues for practice development need to be:

Concerned predominantly with nursing practice

Clearly nursing-led

Grounded in direct patient care

Highly relevant to the particular clinical area/client-group

Agreed by the nursing team to have some significant importance or interest

Compatible beliefs and values of the nursing team

Compatible with the experience, knowledge and/or skill(s) of the nursing team

Project 'pathways'

Each project within a programme of practice development follows the same structure and processes. This group of project participants become a 'cohort' of staff who are able to act as 'agents of change' within their clinical areas. At the same time, they represent their colleagues in defining and influencing the scope of the project. Internal facilitation and regular external supervision support the projects.

In Phase one of the programme, the teams are concerned with exploring the nature of their individual practice development issue. The MHPPDT works with the teams to start developing a range of practice development skills. Early activities include finding and critically appraising any existing 'evidence', which includes research findings, 'best practices', results of local audits, 'opinion leader' evidence and any other body of knowledge which the teams feel might be useful and meaningful for them. At the same time, teams are encouraged to generate ideas and initiate debate within their clinical areas to gain some understanding of what it is that is important to colleagues. They also start to identify their individual and collective knowledge, skills and experiences, as these must be valued as assets within the projects (Biley and Whale, 1996). Additionally, the teams have the opportunity to start exploring those practices which are bound up in ritual and tradition, or are perhaps embedded in dominant and traditional medical psychiatric practice (Walsh and Ford, 1989). They become more aware of unquestioned practices and the potential for new or alternative ways of working. This often alerts the teams to the need for additional learning or skills training.

The teams build on their raised critical awareness, knowledge of relevant literature areas and go on in phase two to evaluate current practice. Each team identifies what type of 'evidence' they will need to collect within their areas in order to describe or measure current practice. In our experience so far, this has predominantly involved the use of staff, patient/client and carer questionnaires, interviews and audits, which largely focuses upon perceptions and experiences in relation to the specific issue. Central to all of the projects is the need to discover the patient/client experience of the practice. Thus, along with other activities, the projects each have several data sets which become the baseline measures against which the practice change can be evaluated at the end of the two years. In response to this information and subsequent new understandings, the teams design the necessary processes for the implementation. For example, this might include designing and organising an educational package.

Phase three of the programme is the implementation phase and will really demonstrate the extent to which the teams have prepared themselves and their colleagues for the practice change. At this stage the information, communication and mechanisms for project decision-making should be well-established. A constant theme running through all projects is the emphasis on communication with colleagues and others to provide the space for feedback, consultation and active participation (Carr and Kemmis, 1986).

The extent to which the teams have incorporated the critical views and participation of their teams in phase one and two will become evident. Further, leading and managing practice development is inherently complex (Kitson *et al*, 1998), it is not simply a task of 'just doing it'. As might be expected, many teams find this phase extremely challenging and require substantial support from within their organisation.

Evaluation occurs in the fourth phase. Here the teams are concerned with critically examining the impact, or not, of their innovation within the clinical area. The baseline data collection tools used in phase two are repeated. It can be expected that many factors may have influenced these 'outcomes' of change, so it is important that the project teams document any changes which occur as a result or 'spin off' from the project and external changes which have impacted on the practice development area (Waterman *et al*, 1995). What is perhaps most important, is that the teams are able to reflect on the many experiences of the project as a whole. The teams are encouraged to value their individual experiences and share them within presentations and a written report, as a full and 'real' account of practice development.

Common themes

The range of knowledge, skills and experiences of all the team members, the internal facilitator and the culture of the individual organisation as a whole influences all individual projects (Kitson *et al*, 1998). We have discovered that there are several themes which seem to be common within the development work of these projects.

Issues of communication and teamwork

These are between themselves as members of a project team; with other members of the nursing team, with other disciplines, and with patients/clients and carers. Importantly, all project teams have had to become much more familiar with the communication channels of their respective organisations in order to publicise their development and promote effective involvement. The need for enhanced team-working and collaboration with other disciplines has been highlighted for most teams at an early stage in their project.

Issues of documentation

The way in which practice is understood and then documented as an agreed and deliberate approach to care. Most projects feel that they need to develop documenting processes to:

- specify the nurses' roles and interventions
- provide a rationale for decision-making
- demonstrate collaboration with the patient/client.

The development of therapeutic or helping relationships

Most teams identify the need to refocus their nursing interventions in response to the information they receive from patients/clients. In addition to a greater general awareness of existing approaches or 'evidence', they often develop a clearer personal and team view of what may, or may not be, helpful or therapeutic to the patient/client.

Organisational structure and culture

All teams have needed to develop a greater understanding of the organisations within which they work. To a greater or lesser degree, project teams have considered the influence of culture and politics on both practice and the management of care. Teams have become increasingly aware of both the potential and existing constraints for the development of nursing practice.

Education and skills

Most teams have found that colleagues often feel ill-equipped to change an area of practice without some additional, specific learning or training. A number of projects have incorporated educational sessions or action learning as a central part of their implementation.

Common challenges

In our experience, several factors operate as common difficulties for project teams. These are:

* the pressures of clinical workload and staffing shortages, which prevent them from taking consistent 'time out'
* varying levels of internal support
* accessibility of supervision
* altering energy levels, particularly in response to clinical demands
* inadequate access to, and training for, information technology
* project team members leaving the clinical team.

Conclusion

We believe that project-based practice development provides the opportunity for nurses to be creative and systematic in relation to their practice. The process of practice development needs to be as evident as the product. However, this type of work does make great demands on the time and energy of all participants, including whole teams and associated colleagues. Extra demands are felt where the level of existing academic skills or project experience is limited. It is crucial that projects are supported by the organisation, and are seen as an investment in both nurse and nursing development.

Early evaluation of this approach (Jackson *et al*, 1999b) has demonstrated that participants feel more critical and are subsequently more confident about their resultant practice. They are more clearly able to articulate a knowledge, theory or evidence base to practice and at the same time set it within the context of contemporary mental health care.

While the projects are always related to every-day practice concerns and might not in themselves appear revolutionary, the process of 'going back to basics', exploring the value base of practice, examining the range of existing evidence and engaging in dialogue with colleagues has illuminated the complexities of psychiatric and mental health nursing.

12

Multi-disciplinary work in mental health

Gail Scothern

Practice development is an area that psychologists have influenced through research findings related to all aspects of clinical work, and through the development of new therapeutic approaches, eg. in dementia care. Service evaluation and development is a familiar area to psychologists who readily involve themselves with questions which relate to clinical practice for their own and other professions. However, in the new NHS climate of clinical governance, with National Service Frameworks, the National Institute for Clinical Excellence (NICE), and the Commission for Health Improvement (CHImp) practice development is taking on a quantitatively, and potentially qualitatively different dimension. While there will be overlap with the material in other chapters, in the developing NHS climate practice development involving and across all disciplines is being driven forward, and it is worth separate consideration of the issues that are raised.

Over the last couple of years in my work within an elderly psychiatric community service I have been involved with initiatives which have been joined by all disciplines, in a management sanctioned clinical effectiveness group. This is undoubtedly a result of the rhetorical shift of government policy speak about management accountability for the clinical integrity of service delivery. The concept of clinical governance (see *Chapter 9*) brings together the philosophy of ensuring high quality care for patients with the mechanisms for ensuring that local services develop quality standards in line with national quality standards (through National Service Frameworks and the National Institute for Clinical Excellence), and that these are monitored locally (Commission for Health Improvement and NHS Performance Assessment Framework). Clinical governance demands a framework that is multi-disciplinary (and possibly multi-agency), being, 'a framework through which NHS organisations are accountable for continuously improving the quality of their services and safeguarding high standards of care by creating an environment in which excellence in clinical care will flourish' (DoH, 1998a).

It must be recognised, however, that the practice of clinical governance at service level – clinical teams analysing and assessing the quality of their services and seeking ways to improve them – will be a multi-disciplinary and often also a multi-agency activity.

DoH, 1999c

Those clinicians, with an interest in the totality of service delivery as well as their own practice, have a new political framework that can support developments provided that the outcome can be expressed in terms of quality, effectiveness and efficiency and, I suspect, provided that it does not challenge existing budgetary considerations, for financial management will have lost none of its significance.

Those who may previously have been reluctant to explore change are required to consider how to demonstrate the integrity of a service; are in a climate where audit, evaluation, research and development are necessary tools in which they need to take an interest. Multi-disciplinary practice development now has the opportunity to develop as a political necessity. Collaboration at senior levels in an organisation is required to focus practice change in line with improved quality and effectiveness within overall service objectives. Practice development is inextricably linked with demonstrating total service quality and developments.

So, if the political agenda is driving a context which facilitates multi-disciplinary practice, and service quality standards; How does multi-disciplinary practice development fit with individual practice development? What sorts of issues will this have an impact on; What can be achieved? And, what are the obstacles?

Fit with individual practice development

Practice development may involve the acquisition of ideas and skills which improves the quality of an individual's approach/technique in clinical practice or in their professional conduct within the organisation. This may or may not involve perspectives from other professional disciplines via example or teaching, and generally has its principal impact at the point of interface with the patient, an impact which accrues to enhance the overall value of service delivered. Multi-disciplinary practice development impacts on service provision in part or all of an organisation; changes in multi-disciplinary practice impact on the philosophy of the service, its operational organisation, and on the shape of what any patient may anticipate in terms of contact with the service. Some level of process change is generally involved.

Issues for multi-disciplinary practice development

In fact there may be very few issues relevant to clinical service delivery where change will have no effect beyond the immediate clinical area or the discipline involved. The following refers to several examples of issues tackled within the framework of a multi-disciplinary clinical effectiveness group in elderly mental health.

For instance, a day hospital in one locality notes a number of attenders over the week who are in the earlier stages of a dementia process.

This group of patients seems to share a discrete set of needs and the nursing staff consider whether developing a day dedicated to assessment and intervention for early dementia sufferers would improve the service they receive, meeting their needs better and encouraging regular attendance. The day hospital can readily make a case for improving the clinical service delivery by making this change with a rearrangement of the timetable and no significant new expenditure. Yet is this really a go-ahead, stand-alone development? Not from a multi-disciplinary, multi-agency whole service perspective.

Consider the implications for re-planning all professionals' time around the service change; some disciplines such as occupational therapy, clinical psychology and indeed psychiatry will have obligations and responsibilities beyond the day hospital to fit around. Consider also the difficulties of making provision to clear a particular day by removing (ie. discharging or rescheduling) those patients attending with severe problems for specialist day care; the sudden demand on social workers for instance to re-organise packages of care, to find suitable alternative day places in existing scarce resources.

Services rarely operate in isolation, and what may initially be a positive idea can create a set of operational problems for related areas and organisations. This may not be an insurmountable obstacle, and it may be that there is some consensus to carry forward change, but it demands an appropriate co-ordinated planning process to carry the decision and move forward the change.

To take another example, an occupational therapy service operates closely with nursing colleagues in community teams.

However, the OT service head is aware that OT staff are working generically, supporting the busy nursing service and working with general referrals to the teams. This leaves no scope to develop their specialist input to the patient group or, indeed, to ensure that all specialist OT assessment is provided to patients across the district in community or inpatient settings. Unmet (probably not identified) need for OT assessment and input is clearly an untenable situation. Yet to withdraw OTs to cover such work has an impact on nursing colleagues handling busy referral rates. This is an occasion when the wider service needs warrant careful consideration with a management acknowledgement of the implications of change or no change.

In another example, a psychologist makes a visit to a ward to assess a newly referred patient. The patient is being nursed on a side-ward and the notes are stamped with information that he is a carrier of MRSA. The ward staff attend the patient without protective clothing. The psychologist bumps into the physiotherapist at his visit, who advises that special clothing be worn.

A dilemma? An occasion where if the organisation has an appropriately maintained database of current policies and procedures, best practice can be readily checked out. Policies and procedures are not the property of one discipline, although at times the procedures may seem most relevant to one or another's practice.

What can multi-disciplinary practice development achieve and what are the obstacles?

As the examples illustrate, a multi-disciplinary, multi-agency approach to issues is extremely important for developing and maintaining the clinical integrity and coherence of a whole service. This will be vital in order for management to meet national frameworks and guidelines, and to demonstrate that clinical governance is being taken seriously.

Multi-disciplinary groups are an arena for integrating information captured in research and audit. Different training backgrounds and perspectives allow for constructive critical appraisal of projects, enhancing the value of work undertaken by, for instance, improving the design of a research project. The multi-disciplinary forum is one where colleagues can learn about each others' approaches, learn about each others' strengths. It is a forum for clinicians to understand the net effects for the service of clinical practice change and of operational change. It is a forum from which clinicians may lobby operational managers when decisions about the operation or administration of the service prove less than sensible for clinicians to work within.

Multi-disciplinary practice development can take place at many levels in an organisation, in settings at ward or day hospital level, within locality community teams. For the greatest impact, key people need to be involved, and there does need to be some operational endorsement of the principle. In order to have overall impact on a service, a multi-disciplinary group which includes the various professional heads of service with links to operational management groups is needed to progress issues effectively. As clinical effectiveness and the general development of quality in clinical services are building blocks of the clinical governance initiative, so that a multi-disciplinary group at such a level can be embraced and afforded some authority. Rather than remaining an area of special interest of a few crusading folk, multi-disciplinary practice development can become integral to a clinical service.

Yet, as with any group or committee undertaking, there are various professional and personal dynamics which will play themselves out, and success depends on working to agreed and shared goals. It also depends on whether busy clinicians will foresee sufficient overall benefit to devote precious time to regular meetings and working parties, as well as on how much administrative time can be made available to assist the work of the group.

Again, the clinical governance initiative can be a useful backdrop, and may provide ammunition for resources.

Direct experience of establishing a multi-disciplinary clinical effectiveness group from scratch, would strongly suggest that there does need to be a lead person to provide continuity of purpose and to maintain communication links with others in the organisation both at management and ground floor levels. Every member of the group will have ongoing clinical and/or operational responsibilities and the person leading or chairing does need to have allocated time and the necessary links to be able to put clinical effectiveness issues on management agendas, as well as to take issues to the group from the management team.

If the work of the group is to drive practice change and to involve staff from all disciplines at all levels, there does need to be appropriate communication across the service; administrative support is essential, if only to assist with accurate notes of each meeting. Each professional on the group should undertake to channel information from and to the group within their particular discipline or to particular localities within the service. Where possible, electronic means of communicating information should be accessed and used; an intranet practice development/clinical effectiveness discussion group would be an ideal mechanism for staff to stay in touch.

The choice of topics or issues to be focused on is crucial. A group at ward or team level may choose to focus on one area at a time, but a group operating for the entire service needs to develop an agenda encompassing issues which can be tackled in various time frames, with short, medium and longer term completion dates. This allows for some fairly immediate feedback for work undertaken as well as allowing members to take on longer term projects slowly. Wider service delivery issues, such as risk assessment tools, outcome measures, user involvement, drug administration procedures, as well as audit and research initiatives are all suitable for the agenda.

Delegation of work to sub-groups and to other staff is essential for reasons of involving as many people as possible in thinking about clinical effectiveness, and netting new ideas and information.

Conclusion

Multi-disciplinary practice development can work. These can be exciting times, with the clinical governance initiative encouraging an approach to clinical practice and service development which at the same time respects particular areas of expertise and breaks down the barriers between different professional groups in the interests of the patient and the wider service delivery issues.

13

A model of joint leadership

Gail Gallie and Lindsey Bowles

This chapter offers two perspectives from two disciplines. It examines the advantages and the difficulties associated with diarchical responsibilities. The subtle difference between physiotherapy and nursing perspectives are evident in the text. *Chapter 14* provides an educational perspective on the practice development unit.

The journey towards accreditation as a practice development unit (PDU) has been stimulating, exasperating, challenging, frustrating, fun, puzzling, enlightening, hard work and most of all a huge learning experience for all involved, particularly for us, its leaders. We offer some insights experienced with the hope that it may assist learning in other similar projects.

The project commenced in 1995 when the combined medical unit decided that multi-disciplinary team working was the key to enhancing the high quality patient care and staff development already delivered in many areas. Staff on the unit sought to use the structured PDU accreditation process as a tool to develop existing examples of excellence in practice, multi-disciplinary communication and shared learning and to disseminate them throughout the Unit. The PDU accreditation process was seen as a tool to develop existing examples of excellence in practice and multi-disciplinary communication and, additionally, an opportunity to share learning and disseminate good practice.

Our aim was to promote good practice through collaboration and reduce any negative effects of a competitive ethos that lacked cohesion and promoted isolated working practice. (The reforms of the 1980s had left a competitive element and this had led to some replication and lack of structured development.) We hoped therefore to reduce replication of unnecessary bureaucracy and promote equality of care across our service.

The accrediting body (The Centre for the Development of Nursing Policy and Practice, University of Leeds) provided an independent critical review of the service against explicit criteria established as being common to centres of excellence. These were achieved with the assistance and support of De Montfort University.

Determining the leadership

The concept of PDU was new and it needed to develop into a tangible reality. Part of that reality was the identification of its leadership. Specified both by criteria and organisational necessity it posed significant dilemmas.

Early work had been accomplished by an enthusiastic core group of fairly senior health care professionals with a shared commitment to multi-disciplinary working and the philosophy of improving patient care through collaborative evidence-based practice. The problem that now faced the group was identifying individuals with the appropriate skills, energy, and commitment for the role, the requirements and demands of which were unknown.

As practice development was at the heart of the project it was seen to be important to have clinically based leadership. However, accreditation criteria stress that PDUs should be developed within existing resources. This would pose particular problems for clinical leaders, requiring the role to be integrated into an established workload. A further challenge for our leadership would be to ensure it was inclusive of the many professions and diverse areas that made up the unit in order to bring about the necessary change in culture. In an acute Trust nursing represents the largest group of health care professionals.

Developing a PDU without a nurse as leader would prove problematic if not impossible. The Trust already has a good example of a nursing development unit (NDU), an organisational system of nurturing and disseminating excellence in nursing. However, their underlying philosophies are fundamentally different. NDUs focus on excellence in care through developing nursing, while PDUs aim to achieve excellence through their team working. Joint leaders were chosen (a practice development nurse [PDN] and a Senior 1 Physiotherapist) because of the concern that the established precedent of NDUs combined with the strong nursing status within the Trust could serve to subvert the multi-disciplinary emphasis of the PDU. It would also assist the perceived problem of issues of representation.

Would joint leadership meet the challenge?

The accrediting body considers the leader of a PDU to be pivotal, providing vision, direction and motivation.

*Leadership is discovering the route ahead and encouraging
and... inspiring others to follow... particularly during times
of change or when the way ahead is unclear.*

Stewart, 1989

Joint leadership raises the potential for confusion around
responsibility, communications and conflicting information; a single
figurehead is more easily recognised. Two people might not share
exactly the same vision for the PDU and strong personalities might
conflict. The decision-making process could become slower, more
difficult, and potentially more expensive. Also, some of the issues
relating to representation of specially or discipline-specific dissemination would remain.

Being unaware of colleagues in similar situations we, as the
elected leaders of the PDU, had to carve our own way, without the
benefit of peer advice or support. It was a risk but one which, on
balance, we considered to be our only viable option. Five years later,
the unit has achieved full accreditation and we are able to celebrate
our joint leadership venture as both a personal and organisational
success.

Initial concerns have been allayed and many of those cautious of
the concept now promote it. Joint leadership is now seen as a viable
and, in some cases, a preferable leadership model for PDUs. Because
the vision led the way for the leaders, and this gradually became
more tangible as we worked through the accreditation process, we
managed to avoid some of the potential problems associated with
shared leadership.

We always tried to ensure that there was equal input into
decision-making and that neither one of us was overriding the other.
It soon became clear that the skills and qualities we each brought to
the role were complementary (or could easily become so). The living
and growing through joint leadership has been a shared professional
and personal experience, warts and all. There is no hiding.

Single discipline professional culture, to inter-
disciplinary culture and leadership

The nurse's perspective

It was both frustrating, and embarrassing that, despite the joint
leadership being publicised throughout the Trust, I was often the

primary contact, particularly for managers and senior staff wishing to discuss or arrange meetings related to PDU issues. This could well have been in part due to an established profile within the organisation and also perhaps informal opportunities which occur at unrelated meetings. To counter this we took the conscious decision to always sign correspondence with both names, alternating the order in which they were presented. Additionally, we always tried to assume that those organising relevant meetings intended both leaders to be present and confirmed arrangements only when both diaries could accommodate them. Gradually this strategy worked although it was somewhat of an uphill struggle.

One personal issue which I found initially hard to deal with was the urge to make unilateral decisions or to give instinctive answers. (In their normal everyday role PDNs are put on the spot about issues as a daily occurrence and I was used and was expected to offer my clinical opinion and judgements). When issues related to the PDU arose in this way I frequently responded spontaneously, using my clinical expertise, educational background and my practical experiences (within nursing). Although personalities will affect this type of response, it was only in relaying these discussions to my co-leader that I gradually learned how individual professional perspectives can differ and how much they can colour our thoughts and attitudes.

As a nurse I have never considered multi-disciplinary working, or the issues of cross-boundary working and shared learning, as anything other than a positive step towards continuity of care. However my previous experiences did not prepare me for the depth of professional parochialism encountered when, during our PDU development, we discussed, usually hypothetically, shared learning and cross-boundary working. The issues raised included a corruption of skills, feared loss of quality, and (worst case scenario) the establishment of generic workers resulting in the loss of total departments or professional groups. During this project I also had to learn to understand the relatively young history of the professions allied to medicine (PAMS), many of which have evolved out of early nursing practice.

It is important to appreciate the double-edged sword of evidence-based practice as there is sometimes scant scientific evidence supporting the intervention of many of the health care professions including nursing. The primary threat to nursing relates to specific practices or skill mix. To suggest providing a health care service without nurses is (almost) unthinkable but it is a real possibility for some of the smaller professions. All health care professions have progressed at differing rates in the various aspects of their 'professionalism', each having strengths and weaknesses. Nursing leaders have often highlighted our potential power, often unrealised or dissipated by our immaturity as a 'profession'. However, the sheer size of nursing makes us powerful in ways which we take for granted, but which we must understand if nurses are to promote true multi-disciplinary working.

Historically, opportunities for service development have arisen via Governmental initiatives. Often bids have a relatively short time frame. These proposals were in our previous model disseminated via the management structure (which included a high proportion of nurses) and were often drawn up between the managers with relevant senior nurses' input. In an effort to ensure multi-disciplinary input, proposals would then be circulated to the team for comment. It was our hope that the PDU would be able to provide a structure which would facilitate the development of these proposals by a relevant multi-disciplinary team from the outset. Planned clinical projects indeed benefited as we moved from a nursing strategy to a PDU strategy. Differing perspectives and additional knowledge, enhanced ideas and skills were harnessed to provide a holistic approach. We were able to ensure resources were appropriately and realistically committed.

The physiotherapist's perspective

From early discussions about the concept of PDUs the ideal sounded very attractive. Once the team agreed to opt-in to the project there was much to be done. The challenge was ensuring that it did indeed become a true multi-disciplinary venture. The enthusiasm shown by some of the clinical nursing leaders for the PDU was obvious. What was not obvious was how this nebulous concept could become a practical reality. The existing culture of the unit did not fully support good collaborative working. Was it possible for this to change? I felt that the only way to influence this process was to become more involved.

As elected leaders neither of us saw ourselves leading from the front. Rather we saw the role as one of facilitating the PDU process by reaching as many of those working at the grass roots of health care practice as possible. In order to do this we had, in effect, to create a new communication and working structure within an existing organisation. As we did this we ensured, at every stage, that there was adequate provision for the multi-disciplinary ethos to be embraced.

We also ensured that our model of joint inter-disciplinary leadership reflected throughout the structure thereby developing future leaders.

As we were drawn more into the role it became clear that we were both accessing slightly different information networks. This served to benefit the development of the PDU and also highlighted subtle differences between the disciplines and their relationship with the wider organisation.

Supported by the Trust the PDU was one of those initiatives that was presented to visiting dignitaries. Rather than dress up for these occasions we often chose to wear uniform. But, uniform or not, I was usually the only non-nurse. This, I feel, helped to draw attention to the wider multi-disciplinary team, and the fact that we were in the business of direct patient care.

I have, at times, been frustrated and dismayed by the apparent disregard and lack of respect shown for the efforts, skills and wealth of experience of colleagues by individuals whose focus is the development of nursing. Often there are others around them as able, if not better qualified for the task they are undertaking. In some circumstances this can lead to a feeling of being undervalued and it can be demoralising to be made aware of projects which have progressed in 'single discipline mode' which then subsequently affect day-to-day multi-disciplinary working at the eleventh hour. This can also prevent effective input into an aspect of care with the net result that there may be inadequate provision of appropriate resources.

I have come to realise that this sort of divisive occurrence is as much borne out of habitual practice and the limitations of decision-making processes, as out of the lack of insight of one profession into the workings of another. The current PDU structure is designed to help prevent some of these problems occurring. It has also been interesting to note that despite the discrepancy in size of the many professions involved in the PDU, representation from nursing has often been the hardest to secure, even with attempts to minimise problems of off-duty by ensuring advance notice of meetings. Perhaps with a potentially smaller voice other staff groups feel the need to make a greater effort to be heard.

Conclusion

Advantages of joint leadership have been identified as being the support offered to an isolated role; the ability to learn and evolve roles together; the ability to utilise the skills of more than one person, and the fact that two can often achieve more together than they can independently (Stewart, 1989). We have been fortunate in experiencing all these benefits as a result of our joint leadership. Problems associated with joint leadership have been identified as being predominantly related to sharing of a power base, dithering or conflicting visions, inequality of time or infringements of roles.

We have learnt that, while we all share fundamental patient focused goals of advocacy, provision of education and high quality care, each profession involved in our PDU has a different culture, background and even language.

As a PDU, this can be a strength but only if, while challenging our assumptions and attitudes, we respect and appreciate our diversity keeping an open mind and thinking creatively. As leaders we have both learnt much and it has not always been a comfortable process. As with any successful partnership there has to be mutual respect, inherent trust, honesty and a shared goal. In our case the vision the PDU represents is dear to both our hearts and a strong motivator.

When we were appointed as PDU leaders our vision was somewhat blurred and our working relationship minimal. The elements required to make the joint leadership successful have developed and we have developed along with it. While we are both proud of our own individual professions and committed to the continuing development and progression of that profession as a discreet entity, it is vital to appreciate that multi-disciplinary working does not of necessity threaten this. We have through our evolution come to realise that the sum of the whole is indeed greater than the sum of its parts.

14

Education institutions and practice development units

Dr Paul Pleasance

This chapter relates specifically to the involvement of the higher education institution (HEI) in the establishment and ongoing development of practice development units (PDUs). It is acknowledged that further discussion and, perhaps, different perspectives would be needed if some of the broader concepts of practice development were to be explored.

The point should be made at the outset that the first reason why higher education institutions (HEIs) need to be involved within practice development units (PDUs) is that the HEIs have the lead responsibility for the education and preparation of the professional practitioners who work in the unit. As Wright (1994) says, speaking of nursing development units, their evolution is, in part, a response to the need to integrate theory and practice as they aim to provide settings where 'the goals of education can be coterminous with those of practice'.

In the multi-disciplinary world of the PDU, then, there is a strong case for the creation of a formal link with the various HEIs (or departments within the same HEI) that run the preparation and continuing education programmes for the full range of professionals within the unit. In reality, it is unlikely and unrealistic that so many departments/HEIs could be directly involved. Thus decisions will need to be made early in the development as to what would be the most appropriate link(s). A strategy would also need to be evolved to ensure that advancements arising from the PDU are communicated to all the departments/HEIs responsible for the local preparation and continuing education of professional practitioners. Such a strategy, designed to focus upon the common ground between the various staff groups, may also be helpful in building bridges between those professional groups, and may assist in the development of collaborative teamwork so essential for the successful life of a PDU (Walsh and Walsh, 1998).

Within the criteria for accreditation of any PDU or NDU, there is likely to be a requirement for involvement of a higher education institution. For example, the Centre for the Development of Nursing Policy and Practice at the University of Leeds makes specific reference within its criteria:

> *'12. Collaborates with Higher Education to formulate theory and to develop staff.*
> *15. Requires a Steering Group which must include: ... the link member from higher education.'*

Furthermore, while not the sole preserve of higher education, most universities would argue that they would be well-equipped to contribute effectively to some of the other criteria such as the development, evaluation and implementation of research. Redfern and Stevens (1998) found that in a survey of 28 NDUs, the links with higher education had been helpful in achieving aims related to research, evaluation and evidence-based practice.

Commensurate with this finding, the University of Leeds states that the link higher education institution has specific responsibility for:

- contributing to the advancement of knowledge
- disseminating, through its student programmes, advancements in practice evaluated by the PDU
- ensuring that such advancements are disseminated to wider audiences through publications, conferences and educational activities.

In the majority of cases, there will need to be some formal acknowledgement of the link and the relationship between the unit and the higher education institution. This may conveniently be implemented through the development and recognition of a memorandum of co-operation; clearly this will have specific features designed to reflect the unique relationship that will be negotiated and developed, but the following example may be seen as a useful starting point.

Depending upon the detail that is built into the memorandum (which will almost certainly need to be scrutinised by the legal representatives of each organisation), there may need to be further supporting documentation that gives detail of how the terms of the memorandum will be put into operation. This will explore who is going to do what, when, and how much of it. Clearly there are different levels of the link; for example, there may be lecturer practitioners/'link lecturers' at the grass roots level who are supported by a designated individual within the HEI who has the authority to commit the university's resources to the work of the

PDU. No one individual within the HEI is likely to be able to demonstrate expertise in the range of educationally orientated activities in which the PDU will become involved. The objective is for the PDU to be able to view the HEI as a resource where the necessary skills may be found – and which can be unlocked by the designated individual.

From what has been already discussed, there may appear to be an assumption (possibly also implicit within some accreditation criteria) that the university is providing a service and is therefore in the role of 'giver'. As such there may, at some stage, be a discussion as to whether there are any explicit financial implications arising from the relationship.

So long as common sense parameters are retained, there are strong arguments that this is very much a symbiotic relationship from which there are very tangible benefits for the HEI. It may thus be concluded that there should be no financial payments involved. These benefits are manifest in the memorandum of co-operation, but they are also clear in the enhancement of the quality of the practice placement experience enjoyed by students. Evidence of this is found, for example, in the finding of Redfern and Stevens (1998) of initiatives such as the development of a student charter within an NDU.

It should also be noted that, particularly in relation to the education and training of nurses, HEIs have for years been trying to find an appropriate focus for the link function for teachers between the academic department and the practice area. With the establishment and ongoing development of a PDU, this role is formalised and has a viable focus. In practical terms there is also a shared commitment to achieving the aims of practice development.

Figure 14.1: Example of memorandum of co-operation

1. This memorandum of co-operation seeks to summarise the agreement between:
   The................ Practice Development Unit, and
   The................ Department of............. University

2. It is agreed that these two organisations will work together in specific areas to further the aims and objectives of each through, inter alia:
   ❖ utilising the combined resources, potential and capability of the two organisations
   ❖ promoting and facilitating the development of staff
   ❖ promoting and facilitating the development of students
   ❖ promoting research, teaching and best practice in health care.

3. The University will:
   ❖ provide appropriate representation on the practice development unit steering committee
   ❖ provide support and advice to the practice development unit's educational and planning activities
   ❖ provide support and advice to the practice development unit's research activities
   ❖ provide access to the research resources of the University
   ❖ contribute to the educational development of staff within the practice development unit
   ❖ contribute to the process of the accreditation of the practice development unit.

4. The practice development unit will:
   ❖ contribute to the education and training of practitioners through appropriate classroom teaching and representation on academic committees
   ❖ contribute to the education and training of practitioners through the provision of practice placements and student supervision that reflect the special characteristics and quality of the practice development unit
   ❖ facilitate access to university researchers and research degree students to the unique environment of the practice development unit (subject to normal ethical considerations and approval).

5. As reflects the nature of the relationship between the practice development unit and the University, these lists are not intended to be exhaustive nor exclusive.

6. Intellectual property rights arising out of this co-operation shall be vested jointly in the two organisations. For the avoidance of doubt, the two organisations agree that intellectual property owned by each at the commencement of this co-operation shall remain the unencumbered property of the owner.

Signed on behalf of the University   Signed on behalf of the PDU

....

Amid the very positive potential benefits and opportunities that working with a PDU can create for an HEI is the rather sobering finding of Pearson (1997). He conducted a study of approximately 80 NDUs within the King's Fund Centre network. Respondents reported ambivalent views of the value of the input from nurse educators and largely negative views about the value of the contribution of nursing academics (seen at the time of this evaluation [1989–91] as being different from nurse educators). The suggestion is that this may be due to how far removed from the unit the HEI is perceived to be. No evidence has been forthcoming to suggest that academics from other professional specialities are viewed particularly differently. What this highlights, yet again, is the need to attempt to narrow the gap. The paradox is that the existence of the development unit, with its implicit aim of attempting to reduce the perceived distance between HEI and practice, has itself highlighted (though not created) the problem.

In practical terms, the day-to-day operationalisation of the input of the HEI into the life of the PDU needs to have some focus – something that colleagues in both camps can get to grips with. Some care and caution needs to be exercised here because it would be easy erroneously to give the impression that the HEI automatically has all the expertise in certain areas and that the practice-based staff have none. This is not the intended impression. It is suggested, however, that the focus of the work of the professional working within practice is likely to be different from the professional working in a pre-dominantly academic environment. In any relationship, it is healthy to attempt to utilise and capitalise upon the strengths of each partner, and it is likely that within the HEI there are staff who have actively sought to develop certain skills. Colleagues focusing primarily on delivering care may, as a result of their different role and work, have less actively cultivated those particular skills. It is perhaps here that the HEI can be most supportive, acting as facilitator in the development of staff in a negotiated and agreed range of activities.

The range of educationally oriented activities will be extensive but may include:

- **Team building activities** – Even on a common sense level, it would seem that good quality teamwork is a crucial foundation stone to the development of a successful PDU. Walsh and Walsh (1998) recommend that the teamwork climate be measured prior to attempting to establish PDU accreditation. Where the level of teamwork appears to be less than satisfactory, staff from the HEI may be ideally placed to facilitate teamwork building activities using appropriate strategies.

- **Teaching and learning activities** – Practice-based staff may benefit from the opportunity to take time out to focus on issues relating to teaching and learning. For example, how to deal with different learning styles and approaches among patients and/or staff and students, the development of educationally sound patient or student-centred teaching materials, packs and resources.

- **Business and strategic planning** – There is no guarantee that academic staff in the linked HEI department will necessarily have these skills; but it is likely that such resources will exist within the HEI as will the skills to facilitate workshops where issues related to business and strategic planning can be addressed.

- **Reflection** – Staff from the HEI may be well placed to facilitate the development of skills in reflection in practice. A useful working definition of the concept of Reflective Learning which appears to be widely accepted is provided by Boyd and Fales (1983), 'the process of internally examining and exploring an issue of concern, triggered by an experience, which creates and clarifies meaning in terms of self, and which results in a changed conceptual perspective'.

The phrase '... changed conceptual perspective' has been effectively interpreted and operationalised by Boud *et al* (1985) as '... new understandings and appreciations'.

Reflection as a learning tool to aid the integration of theory and practice and as a means of enhancing the quality of practice is a prominent theme in the field of health care. Arguably this prominence given to reflection was stimulated by the work of Schön (1983 and 1987).

He asserted that schools involved in the preparation of professionals were failing to produce people who were competent to deal with the real world of professional practice, a deficit which could be remedied, in part, if the education were centred upon developing the ability of the practitioners to reflect. The objective would be to ensure that each new experience faced by the student could, through reflection, become a real learning opportunity.

Scholes (1996) also highlights the need for staff within the PDU to develop similar skills in order to achieve the role transition that is required by the development of the PDU.

An increasing awareness of research among the health care professions has resulted in increasing levels of research skills among practice-based staff. Although with a very small sample (3 units) Redfern and Stevens (1998) found that their hypothesis that research activity would be low in units with no academic links was not supported.

There is some evidence, however, that the focus of research skills (from understanding, awareness and implementation of findings through to submitting formal proposals, making research bids and undertaking projects) can be sharpened by collaboration with HEIs who are likely to have available a wider range of research resources. Academic staff may be able help to facilitate the development of a research and evidence-based culture. As suggested in the memorandum of co-operation, there are also potentially real benefits to the university in that the PDU can provide an excellent and unique research database (subject, of course, to normal ethical and professional considerations).

Scholes' (1996) research makes it clear that staff working within a development unit are likely to be subject to changes in their role. For some there may be the perception that they now work in a goldfish bowl, under the scrutiny of a wide range of interested parties. Others are thrust into a position where they will be required to deliver presentations (whether orally or written) that they had not previously considered themselves equipped to do. The resources of the HEI can be brought to bear to support such colleagues in a range of presentational skills, from writing for publication and preparing conference papers, through to delivering verbal presentations, chairing or managing meetings and even organising conferences.

The PDU is usually a part of a greater whole, one section of a large and complex organisation, subject to and affected by all the politics that are part and parcel of such organisations. Staff within the PDU are likely to find themselves in a position where they have to deal with situations with which they have little or no experience. The HEI, as a comparative outsider, may be helpful in disentangling and rationalising the politics within the organisation in which the PDU is located. In a similar vein, Morrison (1996) highlights in her research that adequate management preparation and academic supervision should be utilised as a means of reducing the risks of stress in NDU clinical leaders.

There is one further issue that warrants mention, a benefit arising coincidentally from the development of close working relationships between the HEI and the PDU.

Recruitment and retention of staff (whether the university's students, or the PDU's qualified and/or unqualified staff) exercises the mind of all corners of the healthcare sector. The 'spirit of enquiry and learning' (Wright, 1994) that characterises the development unit is absolutely consistent with the view of education that is held by educators of health care professionals and the absence of which in practice has been criticised for so long by health care students. In other words, students who experience the culture of the PDU as part of their training are likely to opt to apply for employment there once they are qualified. Similarly, if the HEI has a high profile within the PDU, it becomes the obvious contact point for unregistered staff who may want to progress to professional training and for professional staff exploring their continuing education options.

This chapter has sought to examine some of the issues surrounding the nature and kind of the relationship that can, perhaps should, exist between a higher education institution and a practice development unit. As has been suggested, this relationship should be mutually beneficial and the outcome should be the further achievement of the aims of both organisations. It is not easy, and much effort is required from both parties to make it work effectively. If the outcome is a narrowing of the theory/practice gap, through an organisation where the 'goals of education can be coterminous with those of practice' (Wright, 1994) then that effort is extremely worthwhile.

15

Reflections on a single discipline model

Porsotam Leal

The pharmacy profession is regulated by The Royal Pharmaceutical Society of Great Britain (RPSGB). Students of pharmacy undertake a four-year degree course (recently changed from a three-year course) at one of the sixteen schools of pharmacy, and one year of supervised pre-registration experience in practice. There are about 42,500 pharmacists on the Register of Pharmaceutical Chemists (Council of RPSGB, 1998). Pharmacists are experts on medicines. They are usually in close contact with both patients and other members of the health care team and are able to offer advice on a broad range of issues surrounding the use of medicines. Pharmacists are employed in many different areas of practice. However, the two main areas of work are in community and hospital practice. Industry, academia and Health Authorities (HAs) also employ pharmacists (Mackie,1999).

The dispensing process which is central to the work of the community pharmacist consists of three elements: reviewing and confirming the prescription, filling the prescription, and advising the patient on the safe and effective use of the medicine dispensed. The need for manipulative skills to produce medicines in the pharmacy is in decline due to the growth of the pharmaceutical industry and increased use of manufactured medicines. This decline in the traditional function of the pharmacist is fuelling considerable debate about the future role of the pharmacist. Several models of practice development are under consideration with similar resource implications of skills training and legislative and remuneration changes. Most notable examples of such developments are pharmacist-led clinics (Radley and Hall, 1994), 'brown bag' medication reviews (Goodyer *et al*, 1996) and domiciliary care services (Begley *et al*, 1993). As the delivery of health care becomes more dependent upon successful multi-disciplinary collaboration, increasingly pharmacists see their contributions in terms of overall patient outcomes. An emergent practice model which embraces this focus is pharmaceutical care.

Pharmaceutical care is a concept, proposed by Hepler and Strand (1990), that represents both a major challenge and an opportunity for the future role of pharmacy. There are issues concerning the exact nature of the challenge, whether pharmacists are ready to meet it, and what resources are required to enable opportunities arising from the concept to be realised in practice. These issues ultimately go beyond the confines of the pharmacy profession since it is in the interests of those professions working within the National Health Service (NHS), that full use of the pharmacist's expertise in the use of medicines is made.

This chapter briefly describes the structure and professional activities of community and hospital pharmacy in Britain and then deals with the principal themes just noted.

The structure and function of community and hospital pharmacy

There are about 12,300 community pharmacies in Britain, which comprise independent pharmacies, small chains, large multiples, health centre pharmacies and in-store pharmacies in supermarkets. They provide a network for the distribution of medicines and the provision of health advice to the public and to health professionals. Pharmacy departments in hospitals provide dispensing and clinical services to wards and departments for in-patients and out-patients.

In this chapter, reference is made to community pharmacists, hospital pharmacists and primary care/practice-based pharmacists. Some features of their professional activities, relevant to this discussion about the future provision of pharmaceutical care, now follows. Community pharmacists' core activities involve the dispensing of prescriptions, advising the public on the relief of symptoms and giving advice on prescribed and purchased medicines. Some provide pharmaceutical services to nursing and residential homes, and a few offer prescribing support to local general practitioners (GPs). Significant constraints upon role development include the legal requirement for the personal supervision of the supply of most medicines from pharmacy premises by a pharmacist, restricted access to the patient's full medical notes, persistence of professional tribalism (Beattie, 1995), and the limitations of the present remuneration system.

Community pharmacists in contract with HAs to provide NHS dispensing services are paid by a complex formula which is determined by the Secretary of State after negotiation with the Pharmaceutical Services Negotiating Committee (PSNC). The major part of the settlement is the global sum which is based on prescription numbers. More recently, this has been split to provide payment for additional professional services and for devolution of services to HA level (Jones, 1998). Unfortunately, the sums involved are relatively small and remuneration remains directed to supply (ie. dispensing) rather than service (advisory functions). The role of the pharmacist in self medication is only paid for by a product sale.

The provision of clinical advice about both prescriptions and over the counter medicines is based on partial knowledge of a patient's medical and drug histories.

Hospital pharmacists fulfil a variety of medicines-related functions such as clinical duties on wards, formulary management and the promotion of cost-effective prescribing and dispensing. Some are engaged in specialist activities, for example aseptic services and drug information. Hospital pharmacists have easy access to the patient's medical notes and make a unique contribution to the therapeutic team.

Primary care pharmacists work in GP practices to provide pharmaceutical advice. They have access to patients' medical notes, and are generally non-dispensing. They work closely with GPs to develop practice formularies and facilitate more cost-effective prescribing Other services include the utilisation review of specific drugs, running clinics, such as for anti-coagulant monitoring, and reviewing the medication of patients on complex regimens.

The challenge

The challenge presented to pharmacy by the concept of pharmaceutical care has two elements: first, the nature of the concept itself and the changes to practice it is beginning to promote; and, second, the desired outcomes which the changes are directed towards securing. The rest of this chapter examines each element in turn.

Pharmaceutical care

The term 'pharmaceutical care' was virtually unknown until the late 1980s. It has reached remarkable prominence in less than a decade, and now figures as a key policy imperative on the agenda of many pharmaceutical bodies around the world. Pharmaceutical care has developed in different countries in different ways, depending on the health care system as a whole and the pharmacy culture. The RPSGB embraced the need for a new approach to the provision of community pharmaceutical services in a major report, *Pharmaceutical Care: The future for community pharmacy* (DoH and RPSGB, 1992). This builds upon the central philosophy proposed by Hepler and Strand (1990) in their definitive paper as,

... the responsible provision of drug therapy for the purpose of achieving definite outcomes that improve a patient's quality of life.

In the United States, pharmaceutical care has been redefined several times. Strand and co-workers believed pharmacy needed to move from a product- to a patient-orientation and develop a patient care practice that was documented and evaluated. In contrast to medicine, dentistry and nursing, pharmacy has never had a strong philosophy of practice that binds pharmacists together with one common purpose (Mason, 1999). The current definition is, therefore, based on the premise that pharmaceutical care is a practice in which the practitioner takes responsibility for a patient's drug related needs and holds him or herself accountable for meeting these needs (Simpson, 1997).

According to Cipolle *et al* (1998) traditional pharmacy lacked a foundational practice for its activities, and this contributed to the profession's health care role being relatively unacknowledged by Government and other professional groups.

A practice is characterised by three components:

1. A philosophy (which defines the rules, roles, relationships, and responsibilities of the practitioner).
2. A patient care process (which involves making an assessment to determine the patient's needs, developing a care plan and following up the patient to make sure that his or her needs have been met).
3. A practice management system (which includes all the support required to provide the service to patients in an effective and efficient manner).

Figure 15.1 depicts how providers of pharmaceutical care work. To take care of a patient, an assessment of their needs is required, followed by the development of a care plan and prospective follow-up. The care process follows a model of concordance with the aim of reaching a professional-patient therapeutic alliance (RPSGB and Merck Sharpe and Dohme, 1997). (Concordance is an agreement reached after negotiation between a patient and a health care professional that respects the beliefs and wishes of the patient in determining whether, when and how medicines are to be taken.)

Figure 15.1: The pharmaceutical care process (Cipolle *et al*, 1998)

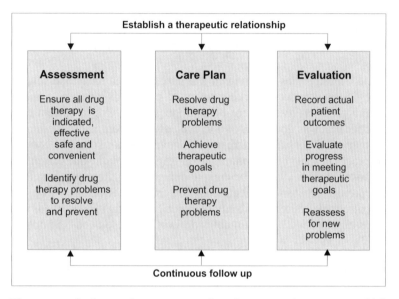

Pharmaceutical care is a structured and systematic process which considers the patient as a whole, therefore preventing pharmacists from choosing one disease or one set of patients. As a generalist practice, its practitioners needed to use the same patient care process. Cipolle *et al* (1998) contrast traditional dispensing pharmacies and those providing pharmaceutical care (*Table 15.1*). For community pharmacists, adding a pharmaceutical care service to an existing product-focused business requires a new orientation that many will find initially difficult to achieve.

The RPSGB is active in the promotion of high quality practice through the development of standards for professional practice set out as an Appendix to the *Code of Ethics* (RPSGB, 1999). The approach used in the document to aid the achievement of pharmaceutical care is to make explicit the underlying principles of pharmaceutical care and then, set standards corresponding to the care process presented in *Figure 15.1*. Professional audit is embraced as an activity through which continuing improvement of professional performance and patient care is likely to be achieved.

Table 15.1: Differences between dispensing products and providing pharmaceutical care (Cipolle *et al*, 1998)

Dispensing pharmacy	Pharmaceutical care
Product business	Service practice
Objective is to bring product to the customer	Objective is to bring the pharmacist to the patient
Decision focus on the (product) business	Decisions focus on the patient
Inventory generates revenue	Patient care generates revenue
Available service supports the product	Available product supports the service
Success measured as number of prescriptions	Success is measured as patient outcomes
Space is organised to display and sell products	Space is organised to meet patient's needs
Records are kept primarily to meet legal requirements concerning drug product	Documentation supports patient care
Frequency of pharmacy use determined by (repeat) prescription service	Schedule for follow-up determined by risk and benefit of drug therapies and needs of the patient
Business is passively sought through the recruitment of patients	Business is actively sought through the generation of prescriptions

The new NHS modern – dependable (DoH, 1997) is a significant change agent for pharmacists' professional future. How viable is pharmaceutical care practice in the evolving health care system?

Desired outcomes

Pharmaceutical care is intentionally aimed at resolving drug therapy problems of individual patients. In Britain, this may lead to savings to primary care groups' unified budgets if the number of drug-related hospital admissions is reduced. Cipolle *et al* (1998) contend that there is a genuine social need to minimise drug-related morbidity and mortality. To effectively meet this social need, practitioners must use a patient-centred approach, which requires that they actually build a practice one patient at a time. Traditional pharmacy remains dependent on prescriptions written by doctors and other prescribers.

Pharmaceutical care involves working with, not for, doctors and other members of the health care team. Pharmaceutical care as a team working concept, linked with other agencies caring for a patient, would greatly assist in integrating drug treatment and therapeutic outcomes into the medical and social models of care currently practised in Britain.

The new NHS modern – dependable (DoH, 1997) strongly

promotes the evolution of a primary care-led NHS and provides the organisational framework for delivering pharmaceutical care within local communities and for the individual patient. Such a service is consistent with the key themes of the new NHS: namely, it should be responsive to need, patient-focused and encompass partnership in provision. Cipolle *et al* (1998) list a number of overlapping foci between pharmaceutical care and primary health care, including patient-centred care, addressing both acute and chronic conditions, emphasising prevention, being accessible to front-line first contact and ensuring integration of care. They go on to argue that specialist services, for example, disease management and drug utilisation review, and practitioner-selected services such as developing local formularies fall outside the remit of either pharmaceutical or primary care.

In England and Wales the medicines management initiative (PSNC, 1998) is different from pharmaceutical care in several important ways. Medicines management focuses on the needs of the community, whereas pharmaceutical care focuses on the needs of individual patients. Furthermore, medicines management appears to reflect the wider political agenda of cost containment. Medicines management demands that its practitioners prioritise their care and target appropriate patient groups (for example, the chronically ill). pharmaceutical care sits somewhat uneasily with each of these aspects.

The underutilisation of pharmacists' expertise, particularly in community practice, must be addressed and the more professionally rewarding and demanding pharmaceutical care practice role embraced. Individual pharmacists and professional organisations are now faced with the task of taking this forward. Can they rise to the challenge?

Meeting the challenge

Smith and Knapp (1992) identify four key issues relevant to the provision of future pharmaceutical care services. These are:

1. Knowledge.
2. Economics.
3. Regulation/legislation.
4. Attitudes.

Knowledge

Although both hospital and community sites are potentially equally suited to the provision of pharmaceutical care practice, individual pharmacists are in a different state of readiness to respond to the demands of pharmaceutical care. The recent clinical pharmacy movement has had most impact on hospital pharmacy. Its practitioners have been able to combine postgraduate education with ward-based experience, establishing themselves as integral members of multi-disciplinary clinical teams. In contrast, few community pharmacists have developed clinical expertise. Many suffer intra-role conflict arising from a lack of congruence between what is learnt in professional training and what community pharmacy practice requires (Barber and Kratz, 1980). This trained redundancy is contributory to the low morale among community practitioners.

In the context of day-to-day practice, only hospital and practice-based pharmacists have access to patients' medical notes. Community pharmacists, on the other hand, are held in a state of dependence by the medical profession, and their aspirations to provide a therapeutic management service are thwarted by this knowledge gap.

Economics

Independent community pharmacy contractors' dependence on the turnover of NHS prescription receipts has steadily increased during the fifty-year lifetime of the NHS. Remuneration continues to be mostly directed to supply (ie. dispensing) rather than service. One consequence of this is the relative reluctance of pharmacy contractors to develop new roles (Jones, 1998). The use of time in pharmacy practice is an important economic concern. Productivity (measured by the volume of prescriptions dispensed) is increasing and, therefore, many community pharmacists are unable to develop professional roles. The employment of pharmacy technicians/dispensing staff in community pharmacies is not universal. The demanding workload of community pharmacists arising from their legal and professional responsibilities, their management roles and the requirements of running businesses is too often overlooked by role development strategists.

Regulation/legislation

The practice of community pharmacy is subject to a number of legal requirements which are designed to regulate the proper distribution and use of medicines. Community pharmacy premises are legally required to be under the personal control of pharmacists. This ties the pharmacist to the premises which severely restricts opportunities for inter-professional activity. Without more frequent and systematic contacts with the health care team, the commonly held perception of the community pharmacist as a supplier of medicines and other products will prevail.

Attitudes

Pharmacists themselves are key to the way the public, other professions and Government perceive pharmacy. What attitudes do pharmacists hold towards aspects of their present and future work? The RPSGB's Council (1995) invited pharmacists in all sectors of practice to participate in 'Pharmacy in a New Age', a consultation process on the future of the profession, affording them an opportunity to share these views. The outcome was the publication of *The New Horizon* (RPSGB, 1996) and *Building the Future* (RPSGB, 1997), which identified five key areas for future development. These include:

1. The management of prescribed medicines.
2. The management of chronic conditions.
3. The management of common ailments.
4. The promotion and support of healthy lifestyles.
5. Advice and support for other health care professionals.

The profession has listed some of the component parts of pharmaceutical care but without putting them together into a practice model. It is clear that pharmacists are seeking to shed their long-standing image as suppliers of drug products (dispensers) for a more professional image based on the premise that they are experts in drug use. In this section, the state of present-day pharmacy practice has been shown to have been crafted by several factors which could be justly accused of supporting the status quo, the most important being the legislative framework for the regulation of medicines and the system for the remuneration of pharmaceutical activities.

Changes, and by implication resources, to achieve the re-orientation of pharmacy to a pharmaceutical care practice model are now discussed.

Seizing the initiative

Perhaps the most frequently mentioned barrier to professional role development is resources, especially time and appropriate remuneration. Dispensing is the most time-consuming element of the community pharmacist's work. Delegation of this core function to properly trained technicians/dispensing staff would be key to solving the problem, but would require some relaxation of supervision. Alternatively, employment of a second pharmacist (particularly relevant in community pharmacies being run single-handedly) may be the preferred option if continuous services are to be provided. Pharmacies will continue their traditional medicines supply function, but this activity will become a component of pharmaceutical care practice. The employment of additional personnel, of course, has major financial implications.

The RPSGB (1999) recently put forward twelve possible alternatives to the current remuneration model. Of these, the 'weighted total capitation' model would seem most responsive to the provision of pharmaceutical care practice. In this model, every patient would be registered with a pharmacy. Payment would be made on the basis of patients registered, but the amount of remuneration would be decided by applying weighting determined by patient need after an assessment of the patient. The Minnesota approach has applied the principles of this model in deriving a 'pharmaceutical care reimbursement grid' (Cipolle *et al*, 1998). The level of payment in this system is based on patient need which is placed into one of five categories. Since the patient is the focus of the payment system it allows payment for all components of pharmaceutical care.

Hepler (1992) urges pharmacists to develop their sense of professional purpose and initiate change at the level of individual practice. He perceives dispensing and clinical pharmacy activities to lie on a professional maturation continuum towards pharmaceutical care. Proponents of pharmaceutical care accept that not all pharmacists will want to make the necessary transition, and estimate a take-up of about twenty-five percent (Cipolle *et al*, 1998). Those likely to accept the new mandate for practice are described by Tann *et al* (1996) as the profession's 'leading edge practitioners' (LEPs).

These individual pharmacists are consistently likely to initiate more actions, be patient-orientated, use a high level of professional expertise, be confident and work effectively with other health care professionals. The researchers suggest that the gap between policy and practice, as well as the time lag in implementation, could be reduced through focusing on LEPs, as key change agents, to pilot and implement recommended changes in practice.

Clinical skills training is core to preparing pharmacists, particularly those in community pharmacy, for a future role in pharmaceutical care provision.

Part-time postgraduate certificate/diploma courses in clinical pharmacy provide in-depth clinical skills through problem-based learning, and instil confidence to collaborate with doctors on prescribing decisions and measuring their outcomes. Participation in such programmes of study would be enhanced through funding to meet locum costs. Individual pharmacists will be expected, along with their professional colleagues from other disciplines, to have appropriate continuing professional development plans in place by April 2000 as part of the Government's clinical governance programme (DoH, 1998a). This initiative will challenge health professionals to demonstrate their professional competence.

The Minnesota project has tested the concept of pharmaceutical care and developed the tools to carry it out (Cipolle *et al*, 1998). The results are promising, but further proof of the beneficial effect of pharmaceutical care on individual patient outcomes is still needed. McElnay (1998) comments that successful future research would require networks of adequately resourced pharmacy research sites in Britain (similar to a multi-centre clinical trial approach), and more robust methods and validated research tools, particularly in the area of outcomes assessment. Maguire (1995) argues that a consortium of parties, including the DoH, RPSGB, PSNC, National Pharmaceutical Association and pharmaceutical industry, should be brought together to provide necessary research funding.

Conclusion

Some of the opportunities and dilemmas which presently face the pharmacy profession in relation to the new pharmaceutical care practice role have been explored in this chapter. By taking the much publicised Minnesota project, areas of opportunity have been identified within the strict approach. It is felt that any attempt by pharmacists in Britain to make a case to adopt the service as part of their professional activity can only be enhanced by the renewed emphasis within the NHS on meeting patient needs and on promoting partnership. Moving from a supply service to pharmaceutical care will improve the standard of patient care, the relationship between the patient and the pharmacist, as well as the relationship of the pharmacist with other health professionals.

However, in seizing these opportunities, the profession also has to address several long-standing dilemmas. These include the constraint on role development imposed by professional and legal requirements for practice, the variation in clinical skills between individual pharmacists, and the product-supply driven remuneration system. These, and other issues will require action by individual practitioners, pharmacy's leadership and Government in order to complete the re-professionalisation process, which began over a decade ago.

16

Professional and legal issues for practice development: safeguards for practice

Keith Todd and Nigel Goodrich

The UKCC, in its position statement on the *Scope of Professional Practice* (UKCC 1992b) states that,

> ... *practice must remain dynamic, relevant and responsive to the changing needs of patients and clients*...

More recently, the Department of Health (1999a) states that the government would like to see the roles of nurses, midwives and health visitors expanded across a variety of settings. Incorporated within this concept is the opportunity to make better use of specialist knowledge and skills, in order to both improve public accessibility to services, and to enhance professional responsiveness to patient or client needs.

Any new development carries with it an inherent risk and the debate surrounding practice development and associated role expansion acknowledges this. Much of the discussion recognises the potential threat to the integrity of holistic nursing or midwifery care (Magennis *et al*, 1999; Castledine, 1994; Denner, 1995), although other authors report that it is perceived as enhancing holistic care (Land *et al*, 1996). The potential threat, however, was anticipated, and an attempt made to pre-empt this by the UKCC itself, in its espoused principles for adjusting the *Scope of Professional Practice* (UKCC, 1992b).

In addition there may be a potential risk to individual patients if the development of any aspect of practice, and its implications, are not carefully thought through. Finally, while patient and client benefit and safety remains the most important issue, there is a need to acknowledge that there may also be a threat to the public's perception of the nurse, midwife or health visitor. There may also, indeed, be a risk to the professional status and registration of individual practitioners involved.

Central to the containment and reduction of these risks is the assumption of professional accountability, and within this concept as a whole there are several distinct professional and legal issues. The exploration and application of these will help to formulate professional safeguards to protect the integrity of nursing care, individual patients and clients receiving this, the professional nurse, midwife and health visitor providing that care and the employer providing the service.

Accountability is the cornerstone of the professional role and practice development. Dimond (1990) offers a useful framework for individual practitioners to view this fundamental issue from both a professional and legal perspective. This provides practitioners with arenas of accountability, including:

- professionally through the UKCC
- to employers through contracts of employment
- legally:
  - to individual patients/clients through civil law
  - to the public through criminal law.

Informed consideration of general principles within these arenas is essential when proposing, negotiating, implementing and ultimately evaluating any form of practice development.

Assuming professional accountability for practice development

Accountability to the nursing profession is essentially through the *Code of Professional Conduct* (UKCC, 1992a), together with the *Scope of Professional Practice* (UKCC, 1992b) and *Guidelines for Professional Practice* (UKCC, 1996b) documents, and supplementary advice papers.

There are perhaps four distinct clauses within the *Code of Professional Conduct* (UKCC, 1992a) and *Scope of Professional Practice* (UKCC, 1992b) documents which relate directly to the general theme of accountability within practice development. According to the UKCC, nurses must always,

... promote and safeguard the interests and well-being of patients and clients.

UKCC, 1992a

And ensure that no actions or omission within their own practice or,

... sphere of responsibility is detrimental to the interests, condition or safety of patients and clients.

UKCC, 1992b

In the context of practice development and role expansion, this general notion is parallelled and re-iterated in the *Scope of Professional Practice* (UKCC, 1992b) document where practitioners are reminded that they must,

> *...be satisfied that each aspect of practice is directed to meeting the needs and serving the interests of the patient or client and must recognise and honour the personal accountability borne for all aspects of professional practice.*

Viewed collectively these clearly demand that any practice development and any associated role expansion is based on a sound, evidenced-based rationale together with very carefully considered benefits for patients and clients. This, in itself, requires that practitioners are aware of current best practice within their individual specialities, have the ability to appraise further research evidence and to translate that into a realistic, achievable form of practice development.

This prerequisite is acknowledged within the Government's White Paper, *Making a Difference* (DoH, 1999a); it states that practice must be evidence based, and proposes a strategy to strengthen the nursing, midwifery and health visiting capacity to both undertake research and to use research evidence to support clinical practice.

Castledine (1994) states that one of the most influential factors affecting the development of clinical practice is the advancement of medical science and technology. This may appear to imply that practice development on the part of nurses, midwives and health visitors may involve the assumption of technical tasks that were once the remit of medical staff, allowing doctors to assimilate and apply the new 'advancements' in medical interventions. These assumed tasks or roles may well be a valid and essential component of any practice development and there is some discussion in the literature (Dowling *et al*, 1996; Tingle, 1997a) regarding who is professionally accountable for the performance of such 'delegated' tasks or interventions. Medical practitioners who, either individually or as a team, negotiate delegated tasks with other disciplines may still be held professionally accountable for those tasks by their own regulatory body (GMC, 1995). It is essential, however, that nurses, midwives and health visitors are fully aware that even if this is the case, they themselves, as registered practitioners, will still be held personally, professionally accountable by the UKCC for the assumption and competent performance of that role.

The report summarising the discussions which took place in the

Heathrow Debate (DoH, 1993a) outlined a slightly broader notion of advancement stating that scientific knowledge and technological innovation would affect where a service is offered and who offers that service. Practice development is, of course, a much broader concept than the simple assumption of roles previously undertaken by other professional groups. It may involve the adoption of scientific knowledge and technological innovation and the subsequent evolution and development of a new service, not previously delivered by any other discrete group within the multi-professional team, such as an alternative therapy, health promotion, counselling or outreach programme. Dyson (1997) makes the point that the medical profession does not own medical and scientific knowledge. She argues that nurses should utilise and incorporate it along with knowledge from other disciplines to augment nursing knowledge in order to underpin practice in a nursing framework. As such, these services could not be delegated to nurses, midwives or health visitors and again each practitioner would be held personally professionally accountable for their own clinical practice within the service.

Whether the area of practice development is the assumption of delegated roles or the growth of a new holistic, comprehensive practitioner role, the issue remains that of competent performance of that role, measured against current prevailing knowledge in the field. This requires, from both a professional and legal accountability point of view, that the performance is measured against an identifiable standard of care. The patient or client must be given the standard of care which would be provided by a reasonable professional following accepted approved practice, while undertaking that task or role (Dimond, 1995a). This is known as the 'Bolam Test' and is the result of a legal case which hinged upon the notion of reasonable practice.

Dimond (1995a) citing a House of Lords ruling in the case of *Wilsher v Essex Area Health Authority*, states that in addition, a patient or client is entitled to the same standard of care whether the work is performed by a nurse or a doctor. Another principle arising from an earlier Court of Appeal judgement in the Wilsher case is that inexperience is no defence to the incompetent performance of a task or role, and a beginner will always be held to the standard of a competent performer of the task (Dowling *et al*, 1996). This has significant implications for practitioners engaged in practice development, whether that incorporates delegated tasks or new service provision. Perhaps the single most important point to be aware of is that the level of competence expected, the reasonable standard, is attached to the role and not to the person undertaking the role. As soon as a practitioner begins to practice a given aspect of care, they are expected to perform it at a reasonable level of competence. These principles have been defined by legal cases establishing legal, liability and accountability, but would also be employed by the UKCC to establish professional accountability.

This has several implications. Practitioners must be aware of their own limitations in relation to both knowledge and skills associated with any proposed practice development, and be prepared to achieve, maintain and develop such knowledge and skills before undertaking new roles. This is reflected in the *Code of Professional Conduct* (UKCC, 1992a) and the *Scope of Professional Practice* (1992b).

This requires a degree of insight and self-concept. Dimond (1995b) makes the point that the inexperienced are not always aware of what they do not know. Professional and legal safeguards require that the innovator of the practice development ensures that an objective assessment of their own, other's or the team's competence, is undertaken to engage in new practice, thereby reviewing current abilities and formulating an education and preparation programme.

Safeguarding of the current service provision may necessitate thoughtful re-adjustment of current individual responsibilities within the team in order to accommodate the resource implications of practice development. Within this, it is essential that inappropriate delegation of aspects of the practitioner's current role, to those not adequately prepared or qualified to assume them, should be avoided.

In turn, colleagues should not be coerced into developing new skills associated with practice development, which are not under-pinned on their part by a sufficient knowledge base and clinical expertise. This should apply equally to both registered practitioners and non-registered practitioners within the team.

It is essential also to be aware that the reasonable standard of competence will not remain static, but will rise as new evidence-based practice evolves. This applies to established 'conventional' nursing or midwifery practice, but ought to come even more sharply into focus when developing and implementing new roles or practice. Tingle (1997b) states that nurses and other health care workers have both a professional and legal duty to keep themselves up to date. He cites a legal case, *Gascoine vs Ian Sheridan and Co* (a firm) *and Latham*, to underpin the principle that health professionals have a duty to keep themselves generally informed regarding mainstream changes in diagnosis, treatment and practice. He suggests that this should be achieved through reference to current specialist journals and leading textbooks within the practitioner's particular field, emphasising again, the notion that updating professional information is essential 'as science and medicine may change and knowledge fades' (Tingle, 1997b) or, indeed, becomes obsolete.

Accountability to employers

Many of the professional accountability issues may have been discussed and considered within the practitioner's immediate peer group or other professional groups within the practice area. Because of the principle of vicarious liability, however, it is absolutely central to any role or practice development, that it is negotiated with, and agreed by, the practitioner's employing body. Dimond (2000) defines vicarious liability as the liability of an employer for any harm caused by employees while acting in the course of their employment. Elsewhere she defines course of employment as 'simply what the employer agrees to the employee undertaking' (Dimond, 1994). Dowling *et al* (1996) state that there is some legal debate as to the definition of course of employment but add that it does allow employers to limit the range of tasks performed 'within the domain of employment'. It is this notion of agreement regarding the range of tasks which affords the practitioner the safeguard of vicarious liability.

It should be noted that this is an additional liability on the employer's part, and theoretically the employer could recover any damages paid to the patient or client, from the negligent employee.

Dimond (2000) states that it is extremely unlikely for an NHS Trust to exercise this right against an employee. She goes on to state, however, that if a practitioner were to act outside their competence they might be regarded as not acting within the course of their employment. The employer would not then be vicariously liable and the practitioner would be personally liable for any compensation to an injured patient or client. Dimond (2000) actually cites the example of a practitioner providing a complementary therapy, acupuncture, without the consent of the employer. She suggests that this may not then be seen as the practitioner's course of employment, rendering him/her personally liable for any compensation paid, should there be any consequent harm to the patient or client.

Further, even if the employer did accept vicarious liability for a practitioner's actions, the nurse, midwife or health visitor might still face disciplinary proceedings, or indeed a UKCC Professional

Conduct Committee hearing, for failing to act within their competence and in line with professional guidelines, (Dimond, 2000).

Dimond (1995a) states that it is essential that practitioners clarify the boundaries of the course of their employment, stating that there are 'considerable dangers' involved if practitioners undertake roles 'without the knowledge and consent of their employers'. It follows from this that any practice development and associated roles should be negotiated with employers and clearly placed within the practitioner's course of employment. Fostering a collegial relationship with employers is likely to enhance the successful implementation of practice developments. This in itself can be achieved by properly assessing the need for the particular practice development, reviewing the evidence base, discussing a structured approach to the change with professional colleagues across the team and negotiating the roles and associated educational and training needs with employers. This could also be seen as the application of two of the principles in *Scope of Professional Practice* (UKCC, 1992b) and of clauses 2 and 3 in *Code of Professional Conduct* (UKCC, 1992a) .

Implementation of the developing role may be undertaken using a range of risk management tools, such as protocols, guidelines, procedures, policies or standards. These will seek to clearly define a boundary for the emerging role in practice and minimise the risk to the employer of non-negotiated practice development.

There is also, however, an onus upon the employer to provide the means for practitioners to develop and maintain the skills to underpin the negotiated practice within these defined boundaries. Lunn (1994) states that, in the context of developing new practice, practitioners should be given the opportunity to both maintain required levels of competence and to obtain new skills.

It might also be advisable for practitioners to consult their individual professional bodies for clarification of the issues surrounding the potential practice development and the implementation of safeguards during the negotiation process with employers.

Legal accountability

In the context of practice development, aspects of criminal law are perhaps less likely to be encountered than those of civil accountability. Dowling *et al* (1996), state that there are two important areas within the civil arena that should be considered.

Reference has already been made to the notion of a reasonable standard of performance, the Bolam Test and the Wilsher judgement. These are grounded within the civil law of negligence. This in itself requires that three components are present before a patient or client can successfully pursue an action for negligence against a practitioner. These include:

+ there is a duty of care owed to the patient or client
+ there has been a breach of that duty
+ there has been foreseeable harm as a result of an action or omission on the part of the practitioner.

A duty of care to the patient or client is an integral part of any practice, be it established, conventional care, or a new development. Any breach of that duty will be measured against prevailing standards of knowledge and competence associated with the area of practice. While foreseeable harm will not be the intended outcome of any practice development, it must be present for practitioners to be found legally negligent. It should be noted, however, that in their pro-active role of public protection the UKCC (1996b) have said that,

> *Professionally, the UKCC's Professional Conduct Committee could find a registered practitioner guilty of misconduct and remove them from the register if he or she failed to care properly for a patient or client, even though they suffered no harm.*

Given that an essential component of civil litigation appears to have been dispensed with by the UKCC, practitioners should be fully aware that any practice development should be carefully considered in order to protect primarily, but not only, the interests of patients and clients, but also their own professional registration.

While this should apply to any area of practice, it may again come sharply into focus where the area of development incorporates non-conventional, complementary or alternative therapies. Indeed, within the same *Guidelines for Professional Practice* (UKCC, 1996b) the UKCC provide explicit advice regarding the relevance and accountability of any complementary or alternative therapy incorporated into an area of practice. This requires that practitioners should carefully consider the underpinning knowledge base and associated assessment of competence.

Both components should be able to withstand rigorous scrutiny when measured against the prevailing reasonable professional standard allied to that particular skill or role.

In the majority of healthcare interventions, the issue of the patient or client's consent to any form of treatment or care is central to maintaining the therapeutic relationship. Unless there are specific exceptional circumstances, evidence that treatment has been undertaken without the patient or client's consent would allow the recipient to seek compensation (Dimond, 1999), even though the patient or client had benefited from it.

Dowling *et al* (1996) citing a legal case, *Re F*, state that battery is committed if a patient is touched without consent. Power (1997) states that the law relating to consent is ambiguous and that nurses need to be aware of the implications of obtaining consent. This, again, should apply to any area of practice. In addition to the general principles of consent, there is, however, an additional element when practice or role development is being considered. Dowling *et al* (1996) go on to say that consent to touching by a specific person or profession will not act as consent to touching by another. This has important implications if the area of practice development involves the performance of roles or skills that might normally be seen as the remit of another discipline other than nursing, midwifery or health visiting.

Dowling *et al* (1996) warn that a patient or client's consent may not be valid if they assume, through the nature of the task, and the way in which the practitioner presents themselves, that they are for example, a doctor or other health care professional normally associated with that role. This is perhaps particularly important if the patient or client appears to be providing implied consent, by submitting themselves unquestioningly to a particular intervention. They advise that there should be an agreed way for practitioners to explain the new role or area of practice to patients and clients, indicating also their professional background and relevant training and experience. From a professional perspective, this may also be reflected in the UKCC's *Guidelines for Professional Practice* (1996b) which state that practitioners must obtain consent for any treatment or care. They go on to state that a patient's or client's decision whether or not to agree to treatment or care must be based on adequate information, in order that they can make up their mind. An explanation of the practitioner's professional background and training might reasonably be regarded as an integral component of that adequate information.

Finally, there is no legal requirement that consent be given in any particular form. It may be provided verbally, in writing or even by implication, such as non-verbal behaviour (Dimond, 1999). Given the particular problems potentially associated with consent and new practice, it may be advisable that evidence of consent is obtained in the written form, particularly where the practice development incorporates new roles, or invasive procedures.

Conclusion

The dynamically evolving nature of health care today provides a significant driving force for practice development. Public protection, however, is central to the government's plans for a modern, dependable health service (DoH, 1999) and is also reflected in professional guidelines (UKCC, 1992a; UKCC, 1992b; UKCC, 1996b).

This necessitates careful management of new roles and new practice development, as potential problems of conflict, resources, education and training and employment issues need to be resolved in order for the maximisation of patient and client benefit to be realised. Careful consideration and rigorous application of safeguards will provide protection from a range of perspectives for patients and clients, employers and ultimately practitioners themselves. Dimond's (1990) framework of the different arenas of accountability also provides a useful structure to consider these practice development safeguards (see *Figure 16.1, p.142*).

Within the context of practice development practitioners must be mindful of the need to be actively involved in the assessment, planning, delivery and evaluation of new aspects of care. Ultimately, nurses, midwives and health visitors must decide the direction and scope of their own practice development, underpinning this with specialist knowledge and a clearly identified role.

Figure 16.1: Safeguards for practice development

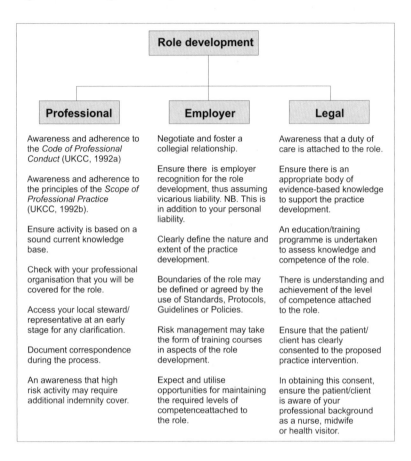

Role development

Professional

Awareness and adherence to the *Code of Professional Conduct* (UKCC, 1992a)

Awareness and adherence to the principles of the *Scope of Professional Practice* (UKCC, 1992b).

Ensure activity is based on a sound current knowledge base.

Check with your professional organisation that you will be covered for the role.

Access your local steward/ representative at an early stage for any clarification.

Document correspondence during the process.

An awareness that high risk activity may require additional indemnity cover.

Employer

Negotiate and foster a collegial relationship.

Ensure there is employer recognition for the role development, thus assuming vicarious liability. NB. This is in addition to your personal liability.

Clearly define the nature and extent of the practice development.

Boundaries of the role may be defined or agreed by the use of Standards, Protocols, Guidelines or Policies.

Risk management may take the form of training courses in aspects of the role development.

Expect and utilise opportunities for maintaining the required levels of competenceattached to the role.

Legal

Awareness that a duty of care is attached to the role.

Ensure there is an appropriate body of evidence-based knowledge to support the practice development.

An education/training programme is undertaken to assess knowledge and competence of the role.

There is understanding and achievement of the level of competence attached to the role.

Ensure that the patient/ client has clearly consented to the proposed practice intervention.

In obtaining this consent, ensure the patient/client is aware of your professional background as a nurse, midwife or health visitor.

Section 3:
The validation and replication of practice development

17

What are the educational opportunities for practice development?

Silvia Ham Ying

There are many educational opportunities that can contribute to gaining the knowledge, skills and attitudes that are necessary for practice development. Before exploring these, it would be helpful to identify examples of the topics about which practice developers should be knowledgeable. This will enable educational needs to be identified so that appropriate educational opportunities can be accessed.

Topics of relevance to practice development

The English National Board (ENB) has identified ten key characteristics of professional competence, based upon extensive research involving managers, patients, practitioners and a range of other stakeholders (ENB, 1991). Practice developers need to be knowledgeable in these areas as they all have relevance to practice development. The ten key characteristics are:

1. Accountability.
2. Clinical skills.
3. Use of research.
4. Team work.
5. Innovation.
6. Health Promotion.
7. Staff development.
8. Resource management.
9. Quality of care.
10. Management of change.

Each of the above characteristics is associated with a number of learning outcomes which amplify the knowledge, skills and attitudes relevant to each key characteristic. These are located in the *Appendix*.

The United Kingdom Central Council (UKCC), in *PREP & YOU Fact Sheet 3* (UKCC, 1995b), has also identified topics of relevance to practice development. These are:

- patient, client and colleague support
- care enhancement
- practice development
- reducing risks
- education development.

In addition to the these topics, the importance of good leadership skills and knowledge is a recurrent theme in professional literature (Marquis and Huston, 1996; Shuldham, 1997; Haworth, 1998). Also of relevance is the development of higher order cognitive abilities such as application, analysis, synthesis and evaluation.

These lists overlap and complement each other. Collectively they provide a useful basis from which educational and training needs relevant to practice development can be identified.

The need for the knowledge and skills identified above has been reinforced not only by the statutory professional bodies but also by the Department of Health (DoH). It is openly acknowledged that the objectives identified in papers such as *The new NHS modern – dependable* (DoH, 1997), *A First Class Service* (DoH, 1998a), *Making a Difference* (DoH, 1999a) and *Saving Lives* (DoH, 1999b) cannot be fully realised without the contribution of nurses, midwives and health visitors and the practice developments in which they will engage.

Relevance of the ENB 10 key characteristics and related topics to practice development

It is important for practice developers to understand the relevance of the topics identified to practice development, so these will be briefly explored.

Accountability

The UKCC through the *Scope of Professional Practice* (UKCC, 1992b), has provided a context for role expansion and practice development. However, the importance of personal professional accountability continues to be stressed. The UKCC (1996b) suggests that,

> ... *professional accountability is fundamentally concerned with weighing up the interest of patients and clients in complex situations, using professional knowledge, judgement and skills to make a decision and enabling you to account for the decision made.*

Practice developers need a good understanding of accountability and the related concepts of responsibility and autonomy. In developing practice, there needs to be clarity about who is responsible for what, to whom individuals are accountable and the level of autonomy that is associated with their role.

Clinical skills

In many cases, practice development requires increased clinical knowledge and skills relevant to the client group of interest. This encompasses what the UKCC (1995a) refers to as care enhancement. Without the appropriate knowledge and skills clients could be put at risk with serious consequences for the patient/client, the employer and health care professionals.

Where care enhancement involves role expansion, it needs to be appreciated that performance will be judged by the same standards used for the professional group that is traditionally associated with carrying out that role.

Use of research

Practice development needs to be underpinned by appropriate evidence. Although it is acknowledged that not all evidence is research-based, research plays an important part in evidence-based practice. Practice developers therefore need an understanding of the different types of evidence that is available, an understanding of the research process and the ability to search, retrieve and critique research papers and other appropriate literature. These skills are particularly important when there are no systematic reviews relevant to the topic of interest.

Team work

Practice development can rarely, if ever, take place as a result of the efforts of one individual. Team work is often an essential component of successful practice development. The composition of the team will vary according to the nature of the development that is being pursued. Within health care, multi-disciplinary team work is frequently necessary even when a particular discipline is leading the development. This is because changes within one discipline can have implications for members of other disciplines. Where the success of the development is dependent upon the co-operation of other disciplines, multi-disciplinary team work becomes imperative. Even when a discipline is not particularly affected by the development, it is good practice to inform them of what is proposed.

Practice developers need to have an understanding of team dynamics and know how to develop and lead effective teams. This is an area in which good leadership skills and knowledge would be beneficial.

Innovation

Practice development is identified by the UKCC (1995b) as one of the areas that practitioners should focus upon in fulfilling their PREP requirements. Flexible, creative and innovative ways of working are associated with practice development and are desirable attributes of practice developers. They need to be aware of sources of practice development ideas. These include:

- government departments
- statutory professional bodies
- professional organisations and trade unions
- employers
- the media – television, radio, internet, newspapers
- service users and their relatives
- peers
- members of other professions/disciplines
- self
- consumer or interest groups literature.

In addition, they need to be familiar with strategies which successfully promote the dissemination and adoption of practice development ideas. The work of Rogers (1983 and 1995) is relevant to this area.

Health promotion

It may be argued that most practice developments are directed at promoting health in its widest context. Frequently, the health promoting activities are directed at patients/clients, their carers and the general public. However, the health of staff is also important though often overlooked. Staff who are unwell, stressed, anxious, de-motivated, change weary and undervalued will not be effective participants in practice development. Consequently, practice developers need to be aware of and utilise strategies that promote the physical, mental and social health of staff, so that they are able to make optimal contributions to the development. Patient, client and colleague support as identified by the UKCC (1995a), is relevant in this context of health promotion.

Staff development

This includes what the UKCC (1995a) refers to as education development. Successful practice development is often dependent upon effective staff development. That is because practice development frequently requires the acquisition of knowledge and skills which are not possessed by the staff who have to participate in the development. Consequently, practice developers need the ability to assess training and development needs, access information about the available resources to meet those needs, and engage in teaching, coaching and motivational activities.

Resource management

Efficiency and effectiveness are still important concepts in the provision of health care. Consequently, the resource implication of any practice development needs to be carefully analysed. In some cases the practice development can occur within existing resources either by utilising staff more efficiently or by re-profiling the workforce so that the skill mix is more appropriate to the developments introduced. In some cases the motivation for the practice development might be to release resources for use in other areas. However, there are occasions when additional resources are required to facilitate practice development. The nature, amount and sources of such resources should be identified. Practice developers will require the ability to develop a case of need, providing evidence of the cost and benefits of the development. They will also require skills of influence and persuasion, making use of relevant opinion leaders when appropriate.

Quality of care

One of the desirable outcomes of practice development is frequently improvement in the quality of the service offered to health care consumers. Practice developers require knowledge of quality indicators relevant to health care, standard setting and benchmarking and the audit cycle. Reducing risks as identified by the UKCC (1995a) is one factor associated with improving the quality of care. Consequently, skills and knowledge of risk assessment and management are required by practice developers.

Management of change

The majority of practice developments are associated with change. Some individuals are resistant to change, preferring the status quo. Practice developers need to be familiar with people's reaction to change, change management strategies and the circumstances under which particular strategies can be most effective in achieving the desired outcomes.

Cognitive abilities

Bloom (1956, cited in Jarvis and Gibson, 1997) identified six levels of knowledge relevant to the cognitive domain. These are arranged in a hierarchy and consist of knowledge of specifics, comprehension, application, analysis, synthesis and evaluation. The lower level cognitive abilities are subsumed within the higher ones, so that knowledge of specifics and comprehension would be subsumed within application, and so on.

Practice developers need higher order cognitive abilities as these are relevant to practice development. In relation to application, they need the ability to use knowledge to underpin practice and to solve problems. Sometimes the knowledge may arise from other disciplines but could be used successfully to guide professional practice and solve associated problems. Analysis is concerned with breaking down issues into their component parts and identifying the relationships between them. In practice development, one needs to be able to analyse the component parts of the development, identifying those most appropriate to contribute to its success. Contributions may be based upon their knowledge and skills, ability to influence and motivate others, ability to provide resources and give permission for the development to take place, and so on.

Synthesis is concerned with drawing the parts together to form the whole. For example, practice developers may read several articles from a variety of authors but should then have the ability to extract the salient points and integrate these into a conclusive statement or view on the state of knowledge relevant to the topic of interest.

Additionally, insights gained from such reading may trigger new ideas or lead to the extension of existing ones which, in turn, could influence practice development.

Finally, evaluation is the ability to judge the value or purpose of ideas, practices and changes. This activity may highlight the need for practice development as existing practices may be inefficient or ineffective and may be failing to achieve the desired outcomes. Evaluation is also an important activity following practice development and the implementation of change. It is important to check that the development or changes have had the desired effects, using standards or other benchmarking procedures in the process.

Educational opportunities for practice development

From the discussions above, it is evident that practice developers require knowledge and skills in many areas. It is now appropriate to explore educational opportunities for practice development in some detail. These include the following:

- In-service/employer-led educational opportunities
- External educational opportunities
- Self-directed educational opportunities.

In-service/employer-led educational opportunities

Health care employers generally recognise the importance of staff development to the provision of good quality care and practice development. While the quality and range of educational opportunities vary from one employer to another, many have some sort of provision in place. It is therefore worth checking with your employer what is available and the procedure for accessing it.

Typical provision includes study days on a range of topics such as accountability, clinical supervision, research, risk management. Skill based courses such as cannulation, cardio-pulmonary resuscitation and venepuncture are also provided. In addition, short courses in counselling, teaching and assessing etc. may be provided.

There are a number of advantages in in-service/employer-led educational opportunities. These include no or low costs to the employee, little or no travelling time, networking with local staff who could provide support and assistance with practice development and the identification of others who are working towards similar goals and with whom collaboration could be mutually beneficial.

Practice developers need to be credible. Appropriate professional and academic qualifications contribute to that credibility. It therefore needs to be acknowledged that some in-service/employer-led educational opportunities are neither professionally nor academically accredited and may not be formally assessed.

This makes it more challenging for such educational opportunities to be accepted as a basis for access to or exemption from aspects of accredited courses. However, evidence of what has been learnt and how that knowledge has been incorporated into practice can be presented in a professional profile and will considerably strengthen the case for access or exemptions.

External educational opportunities

These are both numerous and varied, thus providing individuals with choices appropriate to their needs and circumstances.

External providers of educational opportunities

These include:

* institutions of further and higher education
* statutory professional bodies such as the ENB and UKCC
* professional organisations such as the Royal College of Nursing/Midwifery and the Health Visitors' Association
* trade unions
* societies and associations representing particular interest groups, such as the British Diabetic Association
* government departments such as the department of health
* other health care employers
* social services departments
* publishers, for example, Professional Nurse Conference
* independent providers – individuals or small groups organising conferences and other educational provisions.

Types of external educational opportunities

These include:

* study ½ day/day
* conferences lasting one or more days
* workshops
* short courses
* professional and/or academically accredited modules
* programmes leading to professional and/or academically accredited certificates, diplomas, degrees. These may include ENB post-registration awards, Higher Award and Specialist Practitioner qualification

+ programmes leading to post-graduate diplomas, Masters and PhD.

Typical modes of attendance and access

External providers generally acknowledge the diversity which exists among those wishing to access their educational provision. Consequently, there is increasing emphasis on choice and flexibility. For example, where conferences last for more than one day, a number of conference organisers allow individuals to attend one or more days or the whole conference. This approach allows individuals to pick and mix according to their individual needs and circumstances. Many short and longer courses have both full and part-time modes of attendance. Part-time modes take the form of day or afternoon and/or evening attendance. Some part-time courses are run at weekends or as periodic week long blocks.

Increasingly, open and distance learning materials provide educational opportunities in a wide range of relevant topics. Providers of such materials include the RCN, ENB, Open University, and other institutions of further and higher education (eg. Distance Learning Centre, South Bank University). Several professional journals include distance learning materials, as well as other articles of an educational nature.

With advancing technology, the multi-media are becoming important sources of educational opportunities. These include radio, television, films, videos, satellite transmissions to sites remote from the presentation venue, video conferencing, information technology including interactive programmes and the internet.

Sources of information about external educational opportunities

The majority of external educational providers prepare a prospectus or diary of events which can be obtained upon request. Many will disseminate these to employers and venues of potential customers as part of their marketing strategy. Many provide expanded information in course or event specific information booklets and/or flyers. Individuals who can provide more detailed information about the course or event of interest are normally identified in such materials.

Many educational providers have web pages which provide information via the internet in relation to what they have to offer. Advertising events in journals, newspapers, on the radio and television and through posters and flyers, continue to be a popular means of highlighting educational opportunities.

Approaching educational providers even when they have not marketed their programmes is another way of identifying what is available. Sometimes it is possible to access a central source of certain types of information. One useful example of this is the ENB. It is able to provide information on the different types of post-registration awards which can be undertaken and the institutions which are approved to offer such courses.

Self-directed educational opportunities

Apart from educational opportunities formally organised by internal or external providers, there is a great deal of knowledge and skills that individuals can gain through personal endeavour.

There is a wide range of literature which can be used for self-study. This includes journals, textbooks, open learning materials and publications from government departments, statutory professional bodies, professional organisations, trade unions and societies and associations with specialist interests. In addition, knowledge and skills can be acquired by learning from those who possess them. Opportunities for observational learning can also be sought. Shadowing individuals in certain roles and observing how they operate can provide useful insight into the nature of the role as well as the strategies which work and those which are less effective.

Organising visits to other areas within your place of employment or to external venues which provide examples of good practice or innovations can provide useful opportunities for learning.

The internet provides enormous opportunities for the acquisition of knowledge. Before being able to exploit the full potential of this resource, it may be necessary to improve your information technology skills. This is an example of an area in which assistance may be sought from those more knowledgeable. In using the internet, it needs to be remembered that some information has not been reviewed or validated and therefore should be used judiciously.

Deciding upon which educational opportunities to access

As can be seen, there is a wide range of educational opportunities which contributes to practice development. It is therefore necessary to adopt a systematic approach in deciding which opportunities to access, to avoid the waste of valuable resources by making inappropriate choices. The suggested steps in this decision-making process include:

- assess your educational and training needs – this could be a combination of self-assessment as well as employer-led assessment
- carefully consider your personal circumstances and identify the volume, type and mode of study that could be engaged in without undue stress, and the maximum financial contribution that you could make
- discuss your needs with appropriate individuals within the organisation and establish the contribution that the employer will make in meeting those needs. This could be any combination of study leave, course fees and expenses
- identify the educational activities that will be pursued, taking into consideration your personal circumstances and the resources available to you. Be realistic and do not overload yourself
- ensure that the educational activities chosen are ones which will address specific educational or training needs. Check the content and outcomes of the activities with the providers to confirm that they will meet your needs. If necessary, try other providers to check if they are better able to meet your needs
- avoid accessing educational opportunities without any clear vision of how they will contribute to your personal development.

Conclusion

There are many opportunities for practice development and a variety of methods and providers who can assist practitioners in preparing for the role. Visionary health care professionals will seize these opportunities to improve the care of their patients and clients and enhance their own career prospects.

18

Using clinical supervision in practice development

John Fowler

Clinical supervision is a term that has attracted a considerable amount of interest within health care practice during the 1990s and it has been particularly prominent within the nursing profession. In April 1996 the UKCC issued a *Position Statement On Clinical Supervision For Nursing And Health Visiting* (UKCC, 1996a). This followed a period of consultation with the profession regarding the nature of clinical supervision and if the title 'clinical supervision' was the best term. The general culture at that time for nurses and many health care workers was that once you gained experience and seniority you did not require supervision in the way that it operated with students of the professions. For some people the term 'supervision' implies a 'big brother' approach focusing on inspection and control. However, this was not what the UKCC or the general literature regarding clinical supervision was suggesting. The UKCC position paper (UKCC, 1996a) stated that,

> *The incorporation of the key statements into systems of clinical supervision will allow more effective professional development of nurses and health visitors. This will assist patients and clients to receive high quality safe care in a rapidly changing service environment.*

Although not compulsory the UKCC proposed that all practitioners should have access to clinical supervision throughout their careers. No one model of clinical supervision was proposed by the UKCC. It felt that local needs should influence the development of a model to fit that particular purpose. So, does clinical supervision have anything to offer the experienced health care worker, the clinical specialist, the consultant or practice development nurse?

Consider the following definitions of clinical supervision:

> *Clinical supervision brings practitioners and skilled supervisors together to reflect on practice. Supervision aims to identify solutions to problems, improve practice and increase understanding of professional issues.*
>
> UKCC, 1996a

Clinical supervision involves reflecting upon practice in order to learn from experience and improve competence. An important part of the supervisors role is to facilitate reflection and the learning process.

King's Fund Centre, Kohner, 1994,
Nursing development units

Clinical supervision – a term used to describe a formal process of professional support and learning which enables individual practitioners to develop knowledge and competence, assume responsibility for their own practice and enhance consumer protection and safety of care in complex clinical situations. It is central to the process of learning and to the scope of professional practice and should be seen as a means of encouraging self assessment and analytical and reflective skills.

Department of Health, 1993b

Although the authors acknowledge that there are dangers in trying to give a tight definition to clinical supervision however as a working definition they define it as, 'an exchange between practising professionals to enable the development of professional skills.

Butterworth and Faugier, 1992

Clinical supervision, 'an interpersonal process where a skilled practitioner helps a less skilled or experienced practitioner to achieve professional abilities appropriate to his role. At the same time they are offered counsel and support.

Barber and Norman, 1987

You can see from these definitions that there is no one all encompassing definition of clinical supervision. This is not because no one has given serious thought to the subject or that these definitions are wrong. Rather, it is because the idea of clinical supervision has developed over a number of years from various areas of clinical practice. Clinical supervision for the junior nurse working in a hospital ward will need to be very different from that of an experienced mental health nurse working in the community. If someone tried to develop or impose one model of clinical supervision that was to be used for all types of health care situations and all staff irrespective of their experience, then the result would be something that would be of little or no use to anyone.

How does this help us to explore if clinical supervision has a useful place with staff who are clinical specialists, consultants or those involved in practice development? Well firstly, it tells us that clinical supervision is about reflection on and development of practice. Secondly, it tells us that there is no one model of clinical supervision that is appropriate for all. It is the principles of clinical supervision, eg. reflection, support and feedback that are important for all practitioners, not the model of implementation. Thirdly, we can conclude that the focus of clinical supervision should be determined locally by the staff involved in practice. However, the process does have to be facilitated through various management and professional structures.

Principles of clinical supervision

1. At least two people meeting together for the purpose of clinical supervision.
2. Using 'reflection' to focus upon clinical practice.
3. The meetings are structured and organised.

Although there are differences in the definitions of clinical supervision there are a number of underlying principles that help us identify just what clinical supervision could cover. These include:

1. At least two people are involved in meeting together with a specific purpose of discussing clinical practice. The general assumption is that one of these people is more experienced than the other. There are also examples where clinical supervision involves a small group of people or when both practitioners have similar experiences.
2. Another theme that is common to these definitions is that they not only talk about discussing practice but also reflecting upon it. Reflection upon practice requires structure, focus and objectivity.
3. The conclusions of the discussions and reflections are integrated into future practice by the use of appropriate feedback from an experienced practitioner.

The combination of at least two people meeting together to reflect upon practice requires a degree of organisation or formality that is not a traditional part of health care practice. The more senior and experienced we become the less this seems to occur. We may often meet together to review a patient's care, but this is usually at a level of discussion rather than reflection and tends to focus on immediate problem-solving rather than analysis of previous practice.

If these are the principles of clinical supervision the next question you are probably asking is what is its purpose? If you again review the definitions given earlier you will see that there is not a single purpose to clinical supervision but the possibility of three. These are:

♦ it is a learning process
♦ it is a supportive process
♦ it is a monitoring process.

It may be that clinical supervision as it is developed for one group of practitioners takes on a predominantly supportive process, while for another group the learning process is the most important. Yet for

Figure 18.1: Process of clinical supervision

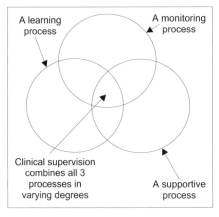

A learning process

A monitoring process

Clinical supervision combines all 3 processes in varying degrees

A supportive process

another group it is a combination of all three that defines the purpose of clinical supervision. For some clinical specialists who work predominantly on their own clinical supervision may offer the opportunity to meet in a small supportive group. A nurse practitioner may value the opportunity to work with a medical consultant in developing a new area of practice. A ward manager may use clinical supervision to provide an opportunity to reflect upon their leadership style with the director of nursing.

So, what is clinical supervision? Clinical supervision is a practice-focused relationship involving an individual or a group of practitioners reflecting on practice, guided by a skilled supervisor. While definitions are useful to aid common understanding, what you need to think through is what are your particular needs and what would clinical supervision have to offer you in your clinical practice. Consider the following areas either for your own practice or for the group of staff that you co-ordinate:

- **The target group** – What are the various groups of staff in your department, ward or unit? Each group of people will have different needs and views on how they would like clinical supervision to work for them. Firstly, identify the different groups that you are responsible for.

- **The purpose** – What is the purpose and function of clinical supervision for each of these different groups of staff?

- **The supervisor** – Who is going to be the supervisor and what are the criteria for appointment for each of the target groups.

- **The ground rules** – What sort of relationship are you expecting between the supervisor and the supervisee? Do there need to be some ground rules?

- **Time involvement** – How much time should be spent in the process of clinical supervision?

- **An agreement** – Does there need to be some form of formal agreement or contract regarding the process or outcomes of clinical supervision?

The target group

Different groups of staff will have different needs and expectations from clinical supervision. If a system that works well for one group of staff is imposed on another group then it is unlikely to be tailored to their specific needs. What are the different groups of staff in your area? Having identified the various target groups within your ward or unit you will then need to identify the particular needs that each of these groups have. Probably the best way to do this is to have each group to meet together and discuss what they see as their needs.

The purpose

The purpose of clinical supervision should be identified and discussed for each of the target groups. Examine the group's needs under three headings.

1. Professional development, which could range from a junior member of staff learning specific skills to the experienced ward sister who wants to develop research skills of finance management.

2. Pastoral support, which might include the discussion of difficult clinical situations or working conditions.

3. Assessment ranging from informal, formative feedback to formal summative assessments, with quality assurance of defined standards falling somewhere in the middle.

The supervisor

The needs of the supervisee and the purpose of clinical supervision need to be matched to the qualities of potential supervisors. The general rule for appointment as supervisor is someone who is enthusiastic to take on the role and has the appropriate experience. The more experienced and specialised you become, the harder it will be to find a more experienced supervisor. You may find a combination approach useful. With a combination approach you could meet with a peer group for general discussion and support. Have some identified time with a professional manager who might focus on your professional development, motivation and leadership needs. Finally, you may want to work with a colleague from a different profession regarding your clinical practice. A number of people may feel that they do not have the confidence, enthusiasm or time to take on another role. This is where appropriate preparation can help the potential supervisor realise that the role can be just as enriching for the supervisor as it is for the supervisee. This perspective may take a degree of 'faith' in the early stages of the relationship but the rewards of supervision should be a real motivating factor once the process is established.

The ground rules

The areas to be considered here relate to the relationship between the supervisor and supervisee, the structure of the supervisory sessions, issues of confidentiality, record keeping. It is likely that there will be some hospital guidelines for some of these issues. Again the important principle is to relate the ground rules to the purpose of clinical supervision to each particular target group. The 'contract' and 'record keeping' for a junior staff nurse is likely to be quite different to that of an experienced ward sister or clinical specialist. However, the principles may be quite similar.

Time involvement

It is important to identify the time involvement as this will help set realistic expectations for the supervisee and the supervisor. The manager, supervisor and supervisee should all agree upon the amount of time to be invested in the process. You need to identify how long and how often. Again this may vary for the different target groups. As a general guideline, the more inexperienced staff will need shorter periods of supervision fairly often, maybe an hour a week. Experienced staff may require a longer session, but not as often, maybe an afternoon every month.

An agreement

The supervisor, supervisee and manager all need to be aware of and agree what is going to happen. If the above steps are worked through, then this can form the basis of a simple agreement on what is expected of all parties involved. A great danger with the implementation of clinical supervision is that there are good intentions in the planning stage, but it never gets beyond two or three sessions because the practical issues have not been thought through and planned for. If you know that your ward gets extra busy at certain times of the year, then how will you safeguard clinical supervision time? What happens when someone moves wards, do they keep their supervisor? You cannot predict all the eventualities, but certain ones you will be able to. The agreement or contract should be used to strengthen the process of clinical supervision, not to inhibit it.

Once you have organised the structure, purpose and ground rules for clinical supervision, you will need to think about the actual sessions or meetings between the supervisor and supervisee. The following guidelines may be useful and can be adapted to suit your situation. The first thing to do is to organise the place where you are meeting so that you are not disturbed. This could mean putting up engaged signs, handing your bleep to someone, transferring the phone and predicting whatever else it is that might cause an interruption. The next thing to do is organise a tea or coffee for you both. Having sorted out the privacy and comfort of the environment and a drink for you both, the next thing to think about is the content of the session. A useful framework for the content of clinical supervision has been taken from the work of Proctor (undated/1986) who identified three areas:

- ◆ formative: the developmental role of supervision
- ◆ normative: the ongoing monitoring, evaluating and assessing role that the supervision might involve
- ◆ restorative: the responsibility for ensuring that the supervisee is adequately refreshed and supported.

It is a good idea to use your first session to discuss together how the sessions could be structured using this formative, normative, restorative structure. In the early sessions it is useful if you include all three areas in each session as part of an informal agenda, although you may want to refine this in later sessions. The formative area is likely to encompass a further three sections of (see *Figure 18.2*):

- Tasks: interpreting cardiac rhythms.
- decisions: which patient do you give more time to?
- reflective practice: bringing to the session a particular clinical incident.

Figure 18.2: The purpose of clinical supervision

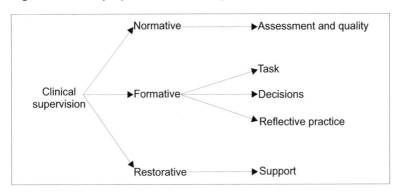

Once you have identified the purpose of clinical supervision, you are in a good position to identify what to say after you have said hello. You can identify the areas that supervision will cover, eg. assessment and quality, development in the areas of certain tasks, decisions or reflective practice, and professional support. If you use these areas as a means of identifying the content to be covered during clinical supervision then the last thing you need to consider is the type of role that you take.

The work of John Heron and his examination of helping relationships forms a useful guide (Heron, 1990). He divides counselling type interactions into one of two classes: authoritative and facilitative. Neither of these is right or wrong, but there are particular times when one or the other may be more appropriate than the other. Each of the classes is divided into three categories, making a total of six categories of possible intervention (see *Table 18.1*).

> **Table 18.1: Heron's six categories of intervention (Heron, 1990 adapted for clinical supervision)**
>
> **Authoritative**
>
> ❖ Prescriptive: A prescriptive intervention seeks to direct the behaviour of the 'supervisee'. This is usually behaviour that is outside the supervisory session.
>
> ❖ Informative: An informative intervention seeks to impart knowledge, information and meaning to the 'supervisee'.
>
> ❖ Confronting: A confronting intervention seeks to raise the 'supervisee' consciousness about some limiting attitude or behaviour of which s/he is relatively unaware.
>
> **Facilitative**
>
> ❖ Cathartic: a cathartic intervention seeks to enable the 'supervisee' to discharge and abreact painful emotion, primarily grief, fear or anger.
>
> ❖ Catalytic: a catalytic intervention seeks to elicit self-discovery, self-directed living, learning and problem solving in the 'supervisee'.
>
> ❖ Supportive: a supportive intervention seeks to affirm the worth and value of the 'supervisee's' person, attitude or actions.

Once you become familiar with this concept then you will have six ways of taking forward the clinical supervision. Some of the direction should be thought out before the session takes place, other responses will need to be more spontaneous.

You should now be in a position to develop and take forward the clinical supervision sessions. The following points summarise the steps to take:

1. Make sure that the place where you meet is private and comfortable.
2. Have a tea or coffee at the beginning of the session.
3. Identify the content to be covered, this may include one or a combination of the following:
    - assessment and quality
    - development of certain tasks
    - development of decision making
    - development of practice via reflection
    - professional support.
4. Think through the various ways in which you can handle the interventions:
    - authoritative:
        ◆ prescriptive

- ◆ informative
- ◆ confronting
- ▪ facilitative:
  - ◆ cathartic
  - ◆ catalytic
  - ◆ supportive.

These ideas are not meant to be a prescriptive model on how to progress your session of clinical supervision. It may be that you take one or two of the ideas and then develop others to meet your needs. Butterworth and Faugier (1992) state that supervision is a personal as well as a professional experience and that it is this human element which allows for the variety of approaches.

There is a delicate balance of informality and formal structure that should form part of a clinical supervision session that is epitomised by the question of should you have an agenda to the meeting? The useful thing about an agenda is that it gives structure to the meeting and lets both people know what is happening. The disadvantage is that the agenda may control the meeting and you may rush through certain areas simply to finish 'the agenda'.

Consider the following sample agenda and see if it could be adapted to meet your need.

Background information

You are the facilitator for a group of six ward sisters who meet together once a month for one and a half hours. The group has been going for one year and has proved to be an informative and supportive group. A basic pattern has developed over the last few months.

- You arrange seven chairs in a circle and put an engaged sign on the door.
- People arrive and help themselves to a drink.
- Sister Smith spends 10 minutes talking about a new dressing that is being used as part of a small research study on her ward. (It was her turn to present the opening session).
- The rest of the group discuss the dressing and also the research trial that Sister Smith is heading up.
- You open the discussion to explore the general issues of introducing new ideas into the ward team.

- The last 30 minutes of the session focuses upon an article that the group is writing. You take a progress report and support any individuals who are finding it difficult.
- You confirm the presenter of the opening session for the next group meeting and set a deadline for a draft of the article.

Most practitioners will not have a great deal of time to sit down and plan an agenda for their clinical supervision sessions. However, time spent planning and collecting your thoughts is a good investment for the busy person. One of the roles of the supervisor is to give direction and focus to the supervisee. A good way of demonstrating commitment to the relationship is for both people to prepare for the session. The balance that needs to be maintained is that the supervisee feels an equal partner in the relationship, it is not you going in a direction that is neither relevant nor interesting to the supervisee. Your experience and knowledge should lead the direction but not dominate it. Both of you should feel that you equally control the situation and the 'agenda'. If there is something more important to discuss then you should feel free to discuss it.

The more specialist and independent practitioners become, the greater is the need for a formalised system of clinical supervision. Whereas staff working in a ward team may have a number of informal opportunities for support, discussion and development, the same cannot always be said for staff working in isolated specialised posts. Clinical supervision offers a way of safeguarding and monitoring of standards, development of practice and support of practitioners. It requires commitment of time, openness to reflect on practice and maturity to admit ones weakness and be willing to learn new ideas and skills.

19

The place of research in the development of practice

Dr Mark RD Johnson

This chapter seeks to argue the case for the involvement of nurses and other health care practitioners in conducting and using research. It discusses some of the problems which arise, as well as giving guidance for critical reading and sources of help in reading and using research. A case study, drawn from life, shows how evidence may be pulled together by a health care practitioner to make the case for a new service, and obtain funding for a health care worker to deliver and evaluate that service.

What relevance does research have for the development of practice, and for the person seeking to deliver health care services 'on the ground'? We all know about those academic researchers who dress up their ideas in a raft of statistics and sub-conditions. Very rarely does a research paper identify where the resources can be located which will permit the practitioner to implement the new developments that they recommend. How often do you read a research paper that helps you do your job, or reads as if its author had worked with real patients? However, the practice of health care is changing, and more demands are being placed on nurses and other health care professionals to read, conduct and use research themselves. In this chapter we shall try to consider what makes 'good' research, and how it might be most useful to those whose duty it is to care. While the main focus may appear to be on activity in primary care, the same messages are true for all branches of nursing, and all settings in which health care is delivered. Indeed, present developments in the organisation of the 'New NHS' in Britain mean that the distinctions between hospital, community and primary care settings are becoming increasingly blurred, and world-wide, health care workers are recognising the essential links between their activities.

It is well known that Florence Nightingale sought to ensure that the improvement of nursing care was based on a scientific and systematic, data-based approach (Roe and Webb, 1998). Similarly, the practice of medicine owes a great deal to the early pioneers of immunisation and public health medicine. Many things that are now 'taken for granted' (such as the germ theory of disease, or the association between malaria and mosquitoes) had first to be 'proven' – or at least demonstrated, by researchers. However, an association between 'science' and 'technology', and a tendency to focus on 'evidence-based medicine' has meant that many aspects of health service delivery and caring have been under-researched and undervalued.

In recent years, this tendency has been increasingly challenged, both by researchers within other (non-medical) professions including nursing, and by the rediscovery in medical research of user-oriented approaches and ethnographic traditions (Helman, 1994; Scambler, 1997).

For those involved in nursing-related activities, the English National Board has laid down a number of recommendations which by now should be everywhere in place and recognised as commonplace (ENB, 1993a; see also Peach, 1999). The board identifies the existence of a cycle of continuous improvement founded on research, development, implementation and evaluation, feeding into and forming part of the education and professional development processes. All nursing education is now expected to be based on research, contain research appreciation and develop research skills.

Nurses, health visitors and midwives need an understanding of the research process, the ability to retrieve and critically assess research findings and literature, and through those skills the capacity to help define research problems, agenda and priorities.

ENB, 1993a, para 3.3.2

With the reorganisation of health care in Britain has come the introduction of a number of new 'service frameworks', including the National Institute for Clinical Excellence (NICE). Many of these have been seen as being a form of rationing, or of limiting the freedom of doctors to prescribe. As nurses, increasingly, also gain the right to prescribe certain items, they will be drawn into this debate, and all health professionals will have to consider the recommendations made by such bodies. Without an understanding of the research process, and the ability to read research critically, these decisions and frameworks will be hard to challenge or appreciate. Similarly, the new framework of primary care groups and Trusts, where multi-professional committees from a variety of health care backgrounds meet to manage health care services, requires a certain amount of common ground between these professions. The language and territory of research provide a means of reaching agreement about key issues.

Clinical governance is the use of evidence-based practice, drawing on 'good' and 'best' practice to improve performance. Research provides the test to ensure that the evidence is robust. The clinical governance approach (see *Chapter 9)* also includes the necessity for personal development through reflection and learning, and increasingly is being seen as a mechanism for collaborative, multi-professional and multi-disciplinary approaches. Good research should meet common standards and facilitate that sharing. Alongside the introduction of clinical governance has been the notion of the HImP, NICE and CHI, that is to say, health improvement plans and clinical standard settings. Research assessment and audit are essential components of these, taking the provider of health care's perspective above that of the individual client to consider the wider picture. All health care workers need to be able to participate as partners in these processes, and to recognise that they have a background in relevant research from which to contribute.

As any health care worker will recognise, their initial training and education only covered what was then known, and thought to be essential to their future practice. As they develop in years and experience, they will encounter new problems (and new diseases, such as the AIDS/HIV infection) as well as learning by reflection about their own needs and experiences. The dilemma is often to recognise how far those experiences are personal and unique, and how far they provide something from which one can generalise. Similarly, there are and always have been, calls to monitor one's work and effectiveness, and to keep and audit records of one's activity. Research is simply the process of testing internal audit processes and reflection against agreed external standards, reflecting on what this may show in more general terms.

There is a lot of poor research around, but we can still learn from it, as long as it is published (ie. made public) with enough data (evidence) to enable informed criticism. The 'gold standard' is often said to be the RCT – a 'randomised controlled trial'. In this model, cases (patients) are allocated randomly to one group or another: one of these groups will be given the new intervention, drug or other treatment, while the control groups are treated in every other way the same. Sometimes, even the 'intervention' may be duplicated – so that the control group may also be given a pill, although it may contain no active ingredients. This should be done, if possible, without either they or their health care professionals knowing which group they are in, so that reactions are not biased by their expectation of change (or no change). RCTs can be arranged so that certain practices, areas or wards in a hospital are given one treatment, and others a different one. The theory is that with a large enough sample population, differences between the groups (such as, to take a theoretical but unlikely example, astrological birth sign) will be very slight, and the main differences in outcome are expected to relate to the intervention. Well established rules have been drawn up for such RCTs, many of which are included in the protocols of the Cochrane Collaboration and other evidence-based practice publications (see websites listed in the *Appendix*). However, some forms of intervention (such as giving pregnant women folate supplements) become so obviously good practice that some trials are abandoned before they are completed. In other cases it proves impossible to conceal what the real intervention is, or it might be thought unethical to do so. In such cases, the researchers have to be extra careful in the way they describe, and think about their study: it is also important to collect enough information to make sure that the 'outcome' is not due to some other process going on at the same time and affecting the two groups differently (as, for example, in two wards on opposite sides of a hospital, one of which overlooks a motorway).

Table 19.1: Aspects of research	
Good research	**Bad research**
Relevant	Exotic
Applicable	Based on ideal settings
Transferable	Unique
Comprehensive	Over-specific
Founded on clear ideas	Over-complex
Justifiable to its subjects	Conducted in secret

For those who are not used to the world of research, it may be difficult to know where to begin. Most researchers, however, are keen to ensure that their findings are widely disseminated and made accessible to those who may act on them. Similarly, many professional associations and those who fund the research have an interest in making these reports easy to find and use. Because of the large number of studies being published, however, it is often helpful to look at summaries and abstracts first, and use these to identify research studies which might be relevant to your own interests. Thus, journals like *Medical Monitor,* the English National Board's *Research Highlights,* or the *Findings* series of the Joseph Rowntree Foundation contain easy-to-read descriptions of recent studies, and give details on how to get more information. Other publications may present a set of reviews and abstracts about a particular topic, and summarise their findings or the differences between pieces of research. Once the practitioner becomes interested and involved, she or he may attend conferences, such as those organised by the Foundation of Nursing Studies, many university research departments, and increasingly, commercial bodies, at which learned papers are presented and debated. From this, they may proceed to read the original papers, or even to conduct small research projects themselves. Once you start to do your own research, you will increasingly begin to read the reports put out by other researchers, to criticise the way they did their studies and to think of things which they might have done differently (or better) or things they might not have thought of. This thinking and testing will, on reflection, have implications for your own practice.

Ideally, health care workers should try and work down that list to get as near as possible to the original source, while realising that the first and last items provide 'ways in', to assess what there might be, and to select what seems to be the most appropriate or accessible as a starting point. The Internet and World Wide Web, while unfamiliar tools to many of those currently in practice, are increasingly becoming accessible, and provide easy ways to keep in touch with research and developments on the wider scene. It is also important to recognise that patients and others in the wider world have access to the Internet too.

Table 19.2: How to access research

❖ Summaries and abstracts – ENB Research Highlights series, JRF *Findings* etc.

❖ Reviews – CRD, Cochrane, Effective Health Care Bulletin, EBP, Bandolier.

❖ Research conferences.

❖ Journals – *British Journal of Nursing, NT Research, British Medical Journal, Journal of Advanced Nursing, British Journal of Occupational Therapy* etc.

❖ Research reports written and published by the researchers, giving full details of their methods and samples as well as their findings.

❖ Internet – which may give access to full-text journals, and databases such as CINAHL, MedLine, National Research Register, EBM etc.

It is good advice to service providers to keep up with your users. It is also important to recognise that theories and fashions change in health care as they do in clothing, music and education. Sociologists insist that we live in a 'post-modern', 'globalised' world where the old certainties and familiar truths no longer provide reliable benchmarks from which to navigate. Research awareness provides a new set of skills which may make this process easier and, indeed, may become addictive.

All research studies seem to end with the words 'more research is needed'. As audit is now recognised to be a cyclic process, where achievement of pre-arranged targets is tested, so research is part of an ongoing cycle of discovery, development and improvement, implementation, and review. It begins with the identification of needs and possibilities, continues through the identification and evaluation of alternative approaches and solutions, to the validation of new interventions and their implementation, and then starts all over again. Once it is established that things can be changed and improved, it is hard to stop looking for better ways of doing them in the future. Research is a key tool in that.

Incontinence and primary care: a case study

Background

Incontinence is still a taboo subject. People are reluctant to discuss it with their doctor. In one study a quarter of the women waited five years before consulting their GP (Norton, 1998). Although over a third of sufferers admit to worrying about their problem, up to two thirds are not known to their GPs.(Thomas *et al*, 1988; Largo-Janssen *et al*, 1990; O'Brien *et al*, 1991) and a qualitative study found that many GPs avoid dealing with the problem (Grealish and O'Down, 1998). There is considerable evidence that incontinence can effectively be treated within the primary care setting especially if a dedicated continence nurse is available (Kelham, 1999). This case study is based upon a proposal which led to the funding of a post for an incontinence nurse to be employed in the 'West PCG' of a Midlands town. A key element in the project was the use of a research-based approach to assess the need for, uptake from, and success of, the new service. All the references cited were located using simple search techniques (available on the Internet) and the library of a school of nursing.

Introduction

One of the first demonstrations showing that incontinence could be managed in primary care came from a well conducted survey in Somerset in 1991, which aimed to measure the unmet needs of patients aged 35–64 with regular urinary incontinence. A postal questionnaire gave a 79% response and showed a prevalence of 16.4% in women and 4.4% in men. Those suffering from stress or urge incontinence or mixed were offered four sessions of pelvic floor exercises and bladder retraining (O'Brien *et al*, 1991).

The evidence indicates that incontinence is a problem that can be effectively assessed and managed by a nurse working to an agreed protocol in general practice. Many of the over 65s (and/or house-bound) are already being seen by district nurses but the under 65 age group are much less likely to be known to hospital and community nursing services, while they do attend GP surgeries for a variety of reasons. For this age range, and the 'active', the success rate of exercise-based incontinence control is better and the social gain implications (eg. work, travelling, shopping etc.) are also significant.

The project nurse would:

- develop ways of identifying unmet needs and encouraging patients to come forward
- assess patients volunteering for the project, using an agreed protocol
- teach pelvic floor exercises and bladder retraining
- follow-up patients (for the audit process assessing the value of the project)
- provide support and training for nurses in other practices becoming involved.

Protocol:

- patients would be invited to attend an assessment at a nearby surgery
- a detailed medical, surgical, gynaecological and urological history would be taken
- urine would be tested using multistix and an MSU taken if positive for nitrites, protein or blood. If either the MSU or further dipstick tests are positive the patient is referred to the GP for further assessment.

Figure 19.1: Adapted from O'Brien, 1991

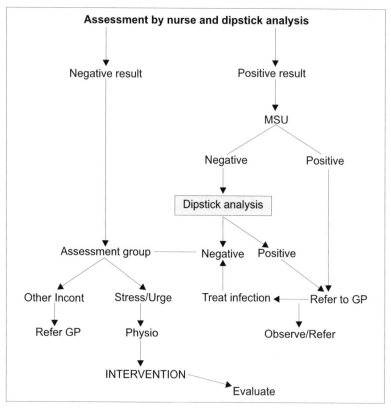

The protocol illustrated in *Figure 19.1* would be used to divide patients into four groups:

- stress incontinence
- urge incontinence
- mixed stress and urge incontinence
- others.

Stress incontinence is diagnosed when the main symptom is leaking when coughing, sneezing, walking or rising from a chair or an inability to interrupt the stream.

Urge incontinence is diagnosed when the predominant symptoms are a desire so great that the person would be wet if they did not get to a toilet or could not hold on for five minutes .

Mixed stress and urge incontinence is diagnosed when no one set of symptoms predominates.

The 'others' include all those with symptoms or signs of voiding difficulty or when the diagnosis is unclear. These would be referred to the GP for further assessment.

Intervention

Pelvic floor exercises would be offered to all patients with stress incontinence, urge incontinence and mixed stress and urge incontinence. Patients with symptoms of urge incontinence would be offered bladder training four weeks after starting pelvic floor exercises. All patients with other diagnoses would be referred back to their GP. The pelvic floor exercises would either be on an individual basis, in a class at a surgery or in the patient's home if they were housebound. In Somerset patients attended four weekly classes which were held in the afternoon and evening, and were then asked to continue 'at home' for a further eight weeks. In the Norwegian study one or two individual sessions were followed by weekly group classes for three months. Clearly, classes are more cost effective and preferred on that basis.

Audit and evaluation

The project will be continually monitored and progress reports will be prepared at two-monthly intervals. Patients (or a sample depending on numbers) will be followed up twelve weeks after their intervention to assess the effectiveness. Audit includes both qualitative, eg. patients' perception of intervention: 'cured, improved, no change, deterioration', confidence to go out etc. and quantitative issues, eg. uptake rates, use of incontinence pads (RCN, 1997) in order to provide an overall measure of the value of the project.

20

Practice development and the role of audit

Denis Walsh

Audit has had a bad press in health care circles in recent years (Oxman, 1995; Sparrow and Robinson, 1992). The term has become overused and, as a consequence, its true meaning has been obscured and, worse still, its original intent devalued. Yet it remains one of the most potent weapons available to clinicians to develop practice if it is applied rigorously.

With the advent of clinical governance in the NHS, audit is making a comeback (DoH, 1998b). This is because it enables the evidence base of care to be appraised in a systematic way and, crucially, challenges clinicians whose practice is at variance with evidence, to change. Sadly, there is abundant proof that even where strong, well disseminated evidence exists, clinicians have remained reluctant to change practice (Peckham, 1991; Iqbal *et al*, 1998).

The dissonance between clinical research and clinical practice has spawned various euphemisms, eg. 'the theory/practice gap', 'ivory tower academia versus coal face realities of practice', and 'a number of research initiatives to explore how the gap can be bridged'. These initiatives have now been systematically reviewed and make for required reading by all clinicians who want to develop their own and others' practice (Thompson *et al*, 1998).

This chapter details the key stages of audit using an example from my own professional background, midwifery. In particular, it highlights the importance of addressing the barriers to change and suggests a number of strategies that can be used to overcome them.

The stages of audit or the audit cycle (see *Figure 20.1*) consist of four elements:

1. The setting of practice standards/guidelines based on evidence.
2. The measuring of practice against the standards/ guidelines in specific pre-chosen areas.
3. The implementation of strategies to address the gap between standards and practice if the standards are not being achieved.
4. The re-measuring of practice to ascertain improvement.

This cycle should be repeated at regular intervals and is analogous to the continuous quality improvement approach of management theories (Morgan and Potter, 1995).

Figure 20.1: Stages of the audit cycle

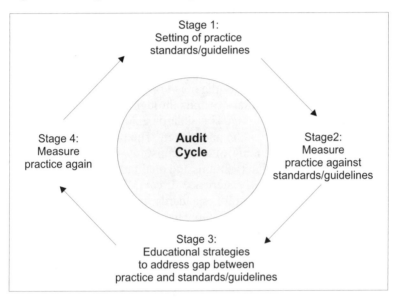

Many audit projects have become fixed at stage two, never moving on to complete 'the audit loop' of stages three and four which, arguably, are the most important phases of audit.

In addition to the four stages, other criteria need to be present if a successful audit is to be completed. These criteria are that the audit should:

- address a known quality issue, ie. sub-optimal care is acknowledged to exist
- be an important area of practice, eg. effect a high volume of patients
- be likely to achieve a qualitative improvement, ie. amenable to problem-solving
- be an area of clinical certainty/consensus
- have explicit, agreed guidelines/standards
- have widespread support of clinicians
- involve multi-disciplinary groups if their collaboration is required to undertake the audit.

Ownership and consensus are therefore key ingredients for undertaking audit.

Within the midwifery context in the UK, there have been few published papers on audit projects that have been robustly undertaken (Odibo, 1997; Brown, 1998) and even fewer where practice has changed significantly (Butler, 1996). Many units are still struggling with the initial step of developing evidence-based standards or guidelines. This was vividly illustrated by the popularity of a local *Handbook of Evidence-Based Guidelines for Intrapartum Midwife-Led Care* (Walsh, 1997) after a national midwifery journal publicised its existence. Over the next six months, 800 copies were distributed to over 75 maternity units throughout the UK.

The development of clinical standards/guidelines is a necessary first step before audit can be undertaken. The process is predicated by a holistic understanding of what constitutes evidence. Clinical trials should evaluate interventions and qualitative methods are best suited to explore client's experience of care. Together their results should inform the setting of standards or guidelines. Clinician involvement in guideline development is mandatory if ownership and consensus are to be achieved.

However, the existence of evidence-based guidelines is no guarantee that practitioner's care will become more evidence-based as Bero *et al* (1998) demonstrate. These authors highlight what is known to date about the effectiveness of interventions to promote change in clinicians' practice. Their taxonomy of methods places the distributions of written materials, eg. clinical guidelines, along with formal lectures, as least effective. Methods of variable effectiveness include the use of influential peers (opinion leaders), local consensus processes and patient mediated feedback and those most effective included educational outreach visits, visual reminders and inter-active educational forums (see *Table 20.1*).

Table 20.1: Taxonomy of educational strategies
Least effective
❖ distribution of educational materials.
❖ lectures.
Moderately effective
❖ feedback of clinical performance.
❖ use of peer respected opinion leaders.
❖ local consensus process of clinicians.
❖ feedback from patients.
Most effective
❖ mentoring of individual clinicians.
❖ electronic or written reminders.
❖ interactive small group educational meetings.
A combination of above strategies

Thompson *et al*'s (1998) review concludes that the outcomes from research into audit's propensity to change practice remains rather equivocal, despite the helpful taxonomy previously alluded to.

They urge researchers to examine the specific barriers to change that operate in clinical practice, which almost certainly will vary from one unit to the next. They suggest a number of barriers that may be more generic in application. These are:

◆ inadequate access to information
◆ clinical uncertainty
◆ concerns about clinical competence
◆ threat of litigation causing practice to be defensive
◆ introducing care that is contrary to conventional practice.

I will refer back to these in the course of detailing the midwifery audit project.

Developing an audit project

The setting for the audit of midwifery birthing practice was a large maternity unit (5,600 births/year) where midwife-led care for low risk women was well established. Four areas of birthing practice, around which there was consensus that current practice was at variance with evidence, were selected to audit. All four areas had been thoroughly researched so there was a strong body of evidence indicating what represented best practice. These were:

1. Intermittent auscultation is the method of choice for monitoring the fetal heart in normal labour as it reduces the risk of operative birth. Routine electronic fetal monitoring should be discontinued (Thacker *et al*, 1999).

2. Pushing in the second stage of labour should be spontaneous as this is associated with less fetal distress and less maternal exhaustion. Routine directed pushing should be abandoned (Thompson, 1995).

3. Women should be encouraged to adopt upright postures for birth as this will result in more intact perineums, fewer assisted births, less pain and makes bearing down easier. Supine and semi-recumbent positions should be discouraged (Sermer and Raines, 1997).

4. Polyglycolic acid sutures are the materials of choice for perineal repair as they are associated with less pain and improved healing. Routine use of catgut should be abandoned (Kettle and Johanson, 1999).

The organisation of care within the unit was based on team midwifery and it was decided to target just one of the midwifery teams so that ownership would be more easily achieved than if a unit-wide initiative were launched. The team was chosen after the midwives responded positively to the invitation to become the first pilot for a birthing practice audit.

The next stage in undertaking an audit project is the writing of an audit proposal. The structure of a proposal has many similarities to a research proposal. It requires objectives, a description of methods and an outline of steps to disseminate findings.

Methods must detail the criteria for sample selection which for this project were:

* women who were judged to be at low obstetric risk at onset of labour
* spontaneous onset of labour between 37 and 42 weeks gestation
* to exclude women who had medical interventions during labour, eg. epidural anaesthesia
* women who had a normal, spontaneous vaginal birth
* only women cared for by the designated team midwives.

Time frames are required for stages two, three and four.

The baseline data of the midwives' birthing practice were collected over three months, followed by one month of various educational strategies to address areas where performance was not consistent with the guidelines. Re-measuring of practice data then occurred over a further three months after which the results were fed back to the team midwives.

Baseline data of birthing practice

Birthing practice in the use of intermittent fetal heart auscultation showed 56% of women had used this method. 8% of women experienced spontaneous pushing during the second stage of labour and 43% gave birth in upright postures. 44% of those who required sutures had Vicryl used for the repair.

As anticipated, there were gaps between what the guidelines promoted and what happened in practice.

Discovering the barriers to change

The identification of the barriers to change determines the choice of strategies to facilitate overcoming those barriers and hence making practice more evidence-based. Therefore an accurate diagnosis of the barriers is critical to success.

Qualitative approaches to ascertaining the barriers are the most fruitful as they yield richer data of individual midwives' perceptions of the problems. Focus group style sessions with the team midwives explored the reasons why practice was not evidence-based. The themes that emerged were:

- lack of knowledge as to what the evidence states about the selected guidelines
- clash between what the evidence shows and individual midwives' experience over years of practice
- skill deficits with adopting new practice techniques
- fear of adopting practices that are not 'main-stream' within the unit
- concern over a risk management backlash if something went wrong.

These concerns mirror those that Thompson *et al* (1998) mention, but additional barriers that proved even more significant were also uncovered and these highlight the importance of doing a local analysis.

It became apparent that how some midwives perceived their role was at odds with key needs of women as elucidated through many recent evaluations of maternity care. These evaluations consistently reveal that women value:

+ information-giving (Kirkham, 1989)
+ control over their own labours (Oakley, 1993)
+ continuity of care (Hodnett, 1998)
+ choice (Green *et al*, 1998).

Some midwives perceived their role as being 'the expert' who knows what is best for their clients and they were reluctant to relinquish any of that control. This barrier can be expressed as a clash of beliefs and expectations between clients and carers.

Discussions also revealed the role of institutional constraints in blocking change. The existence of entrenched hierarchies, both midwifery and medical, within delivery suites sometimes undermined the decision-making of individual midwives who felt constantly under surveillance.

Finally, the physical environment itself militated against change. The clinical decor of a birthing room re-enforced a passive patient role.

Strategies to overcome barriers to change

Some obstacles are far more easy to remedy than others. Access to evidence-based information had already begun to be addressed. In addition to every midwife having a *Handbook of Evidence-Based Guidelines*, the Cochrane Library, Medline and Internet access were all available on the delivery suite. Seminar sessions enabled individual midwives to discuss conflicts between evidence and their experience, eg. some midwives saw exceptions to the guideline about women pushing spontaneously in the second stage of labour. Often women had to be instructed how to do it, in their view. The discussions were facilitated by respected peers (a team leader midwife, the research and development midwife, both practising regularly) who were viewed as opinion leaders within the unit.

Workshops were organised to teach alternative postures for birth and to help midwives assist women to give birth upright. Many midwives had never cared for a woman who had given birth standing. Where possible, midwives observed other midwives who were experienced with these techniques. In these ways, skills deficits were addressed and midwives' confidence enhanced.

Changing beliefs and values around maternity care are profoundly difficult. One approach, which we adopted with some success in this project, was 'personal construct laddering' (Kirkham, 1995). This is a reflective exercise that assists individuals to uncover and articulate their 'baseline values', in this context their attitudes to the client/carer relationship, to childbirth, to the midwife's role.

This can be very sensitive territory, especially for individuals unfamiliar with self-reflection and requires privacy and confidentiality. Therefore, small groups are a pre-requisite for the exercise. Some midwives felt challenged through their participation and became more open to a woman-led rather than practitioner-led approach to labour care.

The difficulties in changing individual attitudes are made even more complex when applied to organisational culture. Institutional constraints are often subtle and subliminal and this is where ethnographic research (in-depth descriptions of an environment and culture), steeped in the qualitative research tradition, can be very useful. Excellent ethnographies of traditional labour wards have been done by both Kirkham (1989) and Hunt and Symonds (1995). They vividly describe the power relationships, the stereotyping of patients and the dominant bio-medical ethos that exist within many. Their studies, though particular to an individual unit, often resonate precisely with one's local environment. Their findings may articulate and describe exactly the culture and enable individuals to see more clearly how to overcome inherent obstacles to change. The midwives in this project were enabled by reading and discussing these studies. It is an excellent example of how evidence from qualitative sources can facilitate the changes in practice required by quantitative research results.

Specifically, the midwives discussed how assertiveness strategies could be used to challenge the status quo and enhance their role as advocates for the women in their care. This impacted on all four guidelines. However, the most potent strategy of all proved to be related to the physical environment.

Since the late 1980s, Home From Home birth rooms (delivery rooms decorated as bedrooms with an explicit natural birth philosophy) have been available for women's use. However, they were increasingly underused in the 1990s for a variety of reasons. Discussions with the team midwives concluded that increasing their uptake by women might have a significant impact in three of the four guidelines. Firstly, continuous fetal heart monitoring was not allowed in these rooms and secondly, the rooms were physically separate from the main delivery suite and, as such, were not under the jurisdiction of senior midwives or obstetricians on the main delivery suite. Thirdly, the emphasis on natural childbirth reinforced the elements of control and choice in childbirth for women. Both upright postures and self-initiated spontaneous pushing in the second stage of labour reflected these themes. The Home From Home environment, because it was exclusively set up for women anticipated to have a normal birth, was at the safer end of the risk continuum and did not attract the scrutiny of risk management as the more 'high risk' delivery suite. For the midwives, this was reassuring and they said they were less likely to practise defensively. The practice of more non-conventional techniques was perceived as easier for similar reasons.

By encouraging women to choose the Home From Home rooms, a number of barriers, including those defined by the context of care, could be surmounted at the one time. Although there were occasionally difficulties in admitting women to this birthing suite, the implementation of this relatively straightforward strategy regarding the environment for birth was probably one of the most effective of all.

Re-measuring practice

All these interventions to facilitate changes in practice were implemented over four weeks and then, after another three months had elapsed, practice was examined again.

Intermittent auscultation of the fetal heart was now occurring in 69% of low risk women. 51% of women pushed spontaneously and 55% of women adopted upright postures for birth during the observational period. 90% of women requiring sutures were stitched with Vicryl.

These results were very encouraging and demonstrate that a well planned audit project can successfully change practice.

Upon reflection, a number of strengths have been identified with the project. Firstly, thorough knowledge of how to develop an audit project enabled realistic goals to be set at the outset and rigour to be applied to each stage. Linked to this was the ownership felt by the midwives who enthusiastically endorsed the selection of the four clinical areas and were motivated to review their practice according to the latest evidence. Of key significance was the elucidating of potential barriers to change, using a focus group method. Midwives found the context of care factors, illuminated so helpfully by ethnographic studies, were a catalyst to both identifying cultural constraints and in overcoming those constraints. Identification of dissonance between women's and midwives' attitudes towards care was helpful for some. The use of influential peers with clinical credibility to facilitate the group activities required to address all the issues was also a significant factor. Educational sessions emphasised participation, inclusiveness and non-judgemental contributions. The team's use of the midwifery birthing suite went up during the audit, illustrating how the environment of care can impact so seminally on practice.

There were also a number of things that would be done differently next time. The data collection period was too short, giving a smaller number of births by the team than anticipated at the beginning of the project. A longer time frame also reassures interested parties that changes in practice are sustainable and not just the 'halo' effect of the observational period. Other educational strategies could have been adopted. The use of written or electronic reminders on notes or workstations and seeking feedback from the women recipients of care are two strategies that will be used next time.

Conclusion

Developments in clinical practice are achievable when evidence and audit are combined effectively. This small project of midwifery birthing practice in a low risk group of women demonstrates that selected clinical guidelines, topical and relevant to midwives, can be audited successfully. Attention to all phases of the audit cycle, in particular the identification of barriers to change and the tailoring of educational strategies to overcome these, are critical to success. Evidence needs to include, where appropriate, qualitative studies that illuminate the context of care as they often enable clinicians to identify and overcome the subtle but often more potent obstacles to change. The clear benefit demonstrated by evidence from controlled trials may never be realised in practice if contextual issues are ignored.

21

Evaluating practice development

John Fowler

The importance of evaluation

The first ward that I worked on as a staff nurse operated a token economy regime for psychiatric patients. These patients had a chronic mental health condition, but had been assessed as having the potential to be rehabilitated into the community. This was in the late 1970s and was part of the early moves regarding care in the community. The ward operated on behaviourist principles, rewarding behaviour that was deemed appropriate and trying to remove the reinforcements of 'inappropriate' behaviour. A number of patients went through this ward learning or regaining social behaviours that would enable them to live in a small hospital flat and then on to houses in the community. This was an ordinary ward in an ordinary hospital, possibly slightly more progressive than some of the psychiatric hospitals of the time, but largely just an ordinary hospital with ordinary staff. I am positive that this ward really did help to rehabilitate a number of these patients and that they achieved a better quality of life than they had previously experienced. In short, I am sure that the ward worked well and, as it was run on ordinary staffing levels, was cost effective. But I cannot prove it because we never evaluated it and we never wrote up and published the experience. This experience is not uncommon to other wards I have worked in, for example, routine recording of electrocardiographs on a medical ward in the early 1970s, managing referrals and discharges as a community psychiatric nurse, and putting various packs in people's nasal cavities on an ENT ward.

Since working in nurse education I have had the privilege to observe others do far more innovative things than my examples. But none of these are exceptional happenings. With very few exceptions most wards or community units that I have observed are not only doing the 'normal' job, but in some small way most areas are trying something new. Sometimes it works well, other times it does not. However, none of my experiences and very few of the others I have seen have been the subject of formal evaluation. Sadly, you have not learnt from my experience and I have not learnt from yours. Until recently the Health Service in general and nursing in particular, did not have a culture of evaluation or even publication of experiences.

If the legacy of the Thatcher government did anything for the Health Service, then it was probably that it introduced a culture that individuals working within the Health Service needed to be able to prove that what they did was not only useful but cost effective. However there are very few nationally led nursing developments. Much of nursing still has a philosophy where innovations and developments happen at ward level, often due to the enthusiasm and leadership of a single person who manages to inspire a team. A recent exception to this has been the recent initiatives from the Department of Health (1993b) and the UKCC (1996a) to introduce clinical supervision. But even with clinical supervision the implementation was often left to individual wards to adopt if they wanted to.

Where then does this leave practice development and evaluation? Well if we are to be honest, practice development is still very much where it was when I was a junior staff nurse in the 1970s. Initiatives developed very much at ward or department level, usually out of existing resources, with little thought of evaluation until the development had been up and running for a year or two. Then someone said, 'we should publish this' or 'we need to evaluate this'. The problem then is that it is probably too late to do any robust evaluation and what is possible requires energy and commitment, which was often centred in one person, who has just moved on to a new job. Am I being too pessimistic here? I would love you to prove me wrong, and I am sure there are a few examples of well resourced and well structured development programmes that not only included the innovation but the evaluation as well. The only nationally co-ordinated approach that I am aware of is the practice development units sponsored by the King's Fund Centre.

The first important point to make is that if practice developments are really going to develop, then we need a national system of trials and evaluations: surgical wards trying out a new dressing, elderly wards trying out a pressure assessment tool, all using the same system of practice and evaluation. The second important point is that while this may be an ideal, and hopefully national leaders will take us in that direction, for the majority of us we will still be working with local projects funded on a shoestring. We therefore need to not only publish our experiences, and this is now happening in a relatively constructive way in the professional journals but we need in addition to build in a philosophy of evaluation from the very start.

If we are going to evaluate practice developments we then need to ask what exactly are we going to evaluate? Is it our views as practitioners, the client's views, the manager's views, patient outcomes, mortality rates? One of the first rules of evaluation is to be very clear about what it is you want to evaluate. You will need to acknowledge that you probably will not be able to evaluate everything. You will also need to recognise that, while you are evaluating one or two areas probably from one perspective, then the practice development may be having other effects that you may or may not recognise. Thus what you will be finding is probably at best a partial evaluation and you must avoid the danger of making claims that cannot be substantiated by your evaluation procedure. Consider the following example regarding the evaluation of hand washing techniques following the use of the toilet by qualified nurses. Review the examples of how this may be done:

1. The nurse in charge of the ward carries out interviews with all her staff regarding their habits.
2. The nurse in charge describes what she believes to be the standard habits based upon her knowledge of her staff.
3. The nurse in charge gives each nurse a questionnaire to fill in and return in person to her after twenty minutes.
4. An independent researcher carries out interviews with the staff.
5. An independent researcher conducts an anonymous questionnaire.
6. A reporter from the local paper asks nurses about their habits.
7. An independent researcher takes a seat in the toilets and openly observes people's hand washing habits.
8. A hidden camera is placed in the toilets (above the wash basins) and is monitored secretly from another location.

Such is the complexity of human behaviour that I would suggest that the only valid evaluation would be the last. It would be interesting to see if ethical permission could be gained for such a study, I doubt it. Absurd as the example is, how many 'evaluations' of clinical practice have you seen published that are based on any of the first seven examples? Sadly, too many. If we are going to evaluate practice we firstly have to be focused on what it is we are trying to evaluate. We must then measure what can be measured and having measured one thing – 'A' not begin to imply that we have really measured 'B' which is something completely different.

There is considerable difficulty in evaluating areas that involve multiple factors. The simplest form of evaluation can occur when a single factor has a single effect. An example of this might be a pharmacological agent that has be developed to act on a specific receptor, which leads to a reduction in blood pressure. However, even with this example, it is rare for one drug to have a single effect. Although there are some aspects of nursing and health care that might be considered in this single cause and effect way, the majority of health care is far more complex and multi factorial. Consider the factors affecting how a patient feels about being admitted to hospital. Have they been on a waiting list for a long time? Have they had a previous admission cancelled? Have they been in pain? Is this an emergency admission? Is the condition life threatening? Is it embarrassing? Does it involve a moral dilemma? How did they arrive at the hospital? Have they come with someone? Could they park the car? Have they left a dependent relative at home? and so on. What about the nurse that is admitting the patient – is this her sixth day on duty? Is she due off duty in ten minutes but someone asked her to admit this patient before she left? Was she expecting the admission? Has she had a chance to read the notes and familiarise herself with the patient's background? Has she just broken up from her partner? Has the ward sister just told her off? Has she just been promoted? Is she the same age, ethnic background, gender as the patient? and so on. These are just a few of the factors that will influence the way a patient feels about being admitted to hospital. Some of the factors are going to be more important for all patients, eg. the life threatening nature of the condition, but others may affect only a few, and others although affecting the majority of patients may not feel important. Equally most of nursing and related health care involves a similar web of complex factors, which are often taken for granted, particularly when we as nurses are exposed to them every day. If we then inject a new factor into the admission of a patient, eg. an admission room or an admission nurse, a reserved car space how can we tell whether it is this new factor that is improving the quality of the admission and not a change in one or a number of the other ones, which we are unaware of? Evaluation of some of the most fundamental roles of health care workers is an enormously difficult task. It is like trying to unweave a tapestry to see why it creates a picture.

You need to be able to see each thread in relation to the one next to it and the effect that changing the colour of one thread will have on others. However, although the picture may look quite simple to start with, once you begin to take it to pieces, you realise how complicated the interactions are. Also the addition of one or two extra threads in certain places may not change the overall picture to any noticeable extent. But the addition of these one or two threads in a slightly different place may change the picture completely.

What is the best method of evaluation?

There is not one method of evaluation that is the best. However there are more appropriate methods depending on the nature of the situation being evaluated. Different methods are also more robust in terms of their ability to predict similar outcomes in future events.

RCTs – randomised controlled trials

This is often referred to as the 'gold standard' of evaluation (Shepperd, Doll and Jenkinson, 1997). An RCT is a longitudinal study in which participants are randomly selected into two groups. One group is given the 'treatment' that is being studied and the other group – the control group, is given nothing. Comparisons are then made between the treatment group and the control group. There are various levels of sophistication of RCTs using double or triple blind approaches, in which the practitioners and researchers are not aware of which group which patient is in, and whether one patient is receiving the 'treatment' or a placebo. If the RCT is well designed with the control and treatment group being as similar as possible with all possible bias being eliminated, and the 'treatment' is a single or easily identified variable and the outcomes objectively measurable, then the evaluative and predictive power of the RCT cannot be bettered. RCTs are used predominantly with pharmacological treatments although there are a few examples of RCTs being used in surgery and other areas (Shepperd, Doll and Jenkinson, 1997).

Before and after studies

Before and after studies (Polit and Hungler, 1995) are another form of longitudinal study in which baseline measurements are made prior to the introduction of a treatment and then similar measurements are made following the introduction. Comparisons are then made between the before and after measurements and conclusions drawn. The difficulty with before and after studies is that other variables apart from the treatment may be introduced over the time period. A number of medical conditions improve on their own over a period of time with no external treatment. If we were to conduct a before and after study on patients with back pain and the treatment was to put a plaster on their back for four weeks, then we would probably find that a significant number of the patients would say that their pain had subsided during the study. We might then claim that our treatment, the plaster, worked! It would not be difficult to exchange the plaster for a slightly more exotic treatment, which could then be marketed and sold. Another before and after study might be to measure staff morale before and after the introduction of a new management system, but again the time interval between the two measurements can be contaminated by a number of other variables. Before and after studies are useful and will often be used to evaluate a new system of health care or approach to nursing.

Provided the results and conclusions are presented within the context of other variables that may have had an influence, then they can be useful in giving general direction and views on what effect the 'treatment' had. However they cannot be used in the same way as well designed RCTs.

Case study

Case studies (Bowling, 1997) focus on a single person or example of what is being studied. They are another example of a longitudinal study that follows a person over a period of time. They may incorporate regular measurements or interviews with the subject. Case studies tend to take a more holistic view of the situation, trying to acknowledge and possibly prioritise the variety of interacting variables that may have affected the person or situation. A case study could take place on a single patient or it could be a case study looking at an out-patient's department or a medical ward. The results and conclusions from a case study approach can be used to give new and more holistic insights into what is happening in a particular situation. What might have been true for the person in the case study might also be relevant to others. What worked in one out-patient's or one ward might be appropriate in another similar area. However, the emphasis must be on the words 'might be relevant' to other similar situations.

Case studies are particularly useful in giving a holistic picture to an event and also in their ability to identify important variables that may have significant influence on a situation. Their strength, which is also their weakness, is that they allow human judgement to interact with a complex multi-variable situation, appreciating the holistic nature of the event as well as identifying possible quirks that may be influencing the situation.

Surveys

Surveys (Bowling, 1997) take a snap shot of a situation often using questionnaires or interviews. Surveys usually begin by identifying a particular group of the population, eg. patients attending a particular out-patient's department, children with asthma, diabetic specialist nurses etc. Using appropriate sampling techniques a proportion of that group is identified. The sample group is then asked certain questions, usually via a questionnaire or sometimes face-to-face. Alternatively, the survey may involve some form of test, observation or investigation, eg. the blood pressure or body weight of the sample group. Provided the sample group has been randomly selected from the population, then the results from the sample can be generalised back to the population. Surveys vary considerably in quality depending upon the degree of randomisation of the sample, the design of the questionnaire or the data collection tool, the implementation of the questionnaire, the response rate, the analysis of the results. They are particularly useful in gaining a general view of a particular group of the population, often being used to gain patient or staff satisfaction views.

If you are going to invest considerable time, energy and resources into developing your practice, then it makes sense that you should also evaluate that practice. In the same way that you will assess, plan and implement the development, you will also need to assess, plan and implement the evaluation. The form of evaluation needs to be included in the initial planning stage.

You may want to include a before and after study or conduct a baseline measure of patient satisfaction. Many of these measurements will be lost once the practice development has started, and if you only begin to consider evaluation once the development is in progress you will find it very difficult to carry out any form of comparative study. Therefore, the first important point in evaluation is to include it in the original planning stage of the development. If at all possible include in this planning stage a person who has a specific remit to oversee the evaluation. If you are coming from a largely clinical background then you may want to invite a research officer or University member to take on this role. The next point is to be as focused as possible in identifying the variable involved in the practice development and the outcomes expected. What is it you want to do and what are you going to measure to see if this has occurred. It is very tempting with any development to jump straight in and get so involved with running the development that you lose track of the wider issues. It is here that a practice development team can give direction, support and feedback regarding the implementation and evaluation of the development. This may involve additional resources, which may be available from within the Trust or may be available from outside agencies. A practice development team will be in a far stronger position to access additional resources than someone working in isolation. Selection procedures for any additional funding, although time-consuming, are likely to focus your thoughts on both the form of practice development and the style of evaluation.

If your practice development is already underway and you did not incorporate an evaluation strategy from the start, then you can still undertake some form of evaluation. This may be a survey of satisfaction or a measure of patient throughput or waiting times etc. Some of these measures may be comparable to similar national statistics. Even at this stage you would be well advised to engage the advice of an independent person to act as evaluator. Any evaluation that is undertaken by the person implementing the development is likely to be seen as being biased, even if the evaluation was objectively undertaken.

Having undertaken some innovative form of practice development, and hopefully having undertaken some form of evaluation of the development, you must then publish your results. Again there are benefits here of a team approach. If you have implemented and evaluated the practice development yourself, you will probably have run out of energy by the time you have some results worth publishing. If you have worked as part of a team, with different people having responsibility for different aspects of the development, then when you come to publication the team will act as a motivator.

Publication in appropriate journals and sharing of experiences at conferences are both a little daunting if you work alone and have not experienced this form of presentation before. Working within a team which incorporates people with different skills and experiences can help take a development through from planning, implementation, evaluation and publication of results.

References

Alty A (1997) Nurse's learning experience and expressed opinion regarding seclusion practice within one NHS Trust. *J Adv Nurs* **25**: 786–93

Anderson N, West M (1994) *Team Climate Inventory Questionnaire*. NFER-Nelson, Windsor

Andrews M (1996) Using reflection to develop clinical expertise. *Br J Nurs* **5**(8): 508–13

Arygris C, Schön D (1974) *Theory in Practice: Increasing professional effectiveness*. Addison Wesley, Massachusetts

Atkins JM (1993) Developments in the philosophy/sociology of science and action research. *Educational Action Research* **1**: 187–188

Atkins S, Murphy K (1993) Reflection: A review of the literature. *J Adv Nurs* **18**: 1188–92

Australian/New Zealand Standard 4360 (1999) Risk management, noted in Governance in The New NHS. Controls Assurance Statements 1999/ 2000: Risk Management and Organisational Controls. *Department of Health,* 21 May 1999

Baly M (ed) (1995) *Nursing and Social Change*. Routledge, London

Barber JH, Kratz CR (1980) *Towards Team Care*. Churchill Livingstone, London

Barber P, Norman I (1987) Skills in supervision. *Nurs Times* **14**: 56–7

Barton R (1959) *Institutional Neurosis*. John Wright, Bristol

Beattie A (1995) War and peace among the health tribes. In: Soothffi K, Mackay L, Webb C (eds) *Interprofessional Relations In Health Care*. Edward Arnold, London

Beer M (1980) *Organisation Change and Development: A Systems View*. Goodyear, Santa Monica

Begley S, Wilhamson V, Hodges N, Livingstone C (1993) Provision of domicilliary pharmacy services by community pharmacists. *Pharma J Suppl* R32

Belbin RM (1981) *Management teams – Why they succeed or fail*. Heinemann, London

Benner P, Tanner C (1987) How expert nurses use intuition. *Am J Nurs* January: 23–31

Benner P (1984) *From Novice to Expert: Excellence and power in clinical nursing practice*. Addison-Wesley, California

Bender MP, Cheston R (1997) Inhabitants of a lost kingdom: a model of the subjective experiences of dementia. *Ageing and Society* **17**: 513–32

Bennis WG, Benne KD, Chin R (1976) *The Planning of Change.* 3rd edn. Holt Rinehart & Winston, Orlando

Beresford L (1998) *Putting Our Best Feet Forward: A pathway to excellent services.* Huddersfield NHS Trust, Huddersfield

Bergman R (ed) (1990) *Nursing Research for Nursing Practice: An international perspective.* Chapman and Hall, London

Bero L, Grilli R, Grimshaw M, Harvey E *et al* (1998) Closing the gap between research and practice: an overview of systematic reviews of interventions to promote the implementation of research findings. *Br Med J* 317: 368–465

Biddington WE (1996) A proactive approach to maximizing training. *Elderly Care* 8(6): 8–11

Biley A, Whale Z (1996) Feminist approaches to change and nursing development. *J Clin Nurs* 5: 159–63

Boud D, Keogh R, Walker D (1985) *Reflection: Turning Experience into Learning.* Kogan Page, London

Boyd EM, Fales AW (1983) Reflective learning: key to learning from experience. *J Humanistic Psych* 23(2): 99–117

Bolam v Friern Hospital Management Committee [1957] 2 All ER 118. In: Dimond B (1995a) The scope of professional practice and the accident & emergency nurse. *Accid Emerg Nurs* 3: 105–7

Bowling A (1997) *Research Methods in Health.* Open University Press, Milton Keynes

Brager G, Specht, H, Torcztner JL (1987) *Community Organising.* 2nd edn. Columbia University Press, New York

Breeze JA, Repper J (1998) Struggling for control: the care experiences of 'difficult' patients in mental health services. *J Adv Nurs* 28(6): 1301–11

Brooks EL, Fletcher K, Wahlstedt PA (1998) Focus group interviews: assessment of continuing education needs for the advanced practice nurse. *J Cont Educ Nurs* 29(1): 27–31, 46–7

Brown L (1998) The tide has turned: audit of water birth. *Br J Midwifery* 6(4): 236–43

Butler J (1996) New breastfeeding standards used as tool of change. *Nurs Times* 92(23): 40–2

Butterworth T, Faugier J (1992) *Clinical Supervision and Mentorship in Nursing.* Chapman and Hall, London

Butterworth T (1999) Educating Nurses: Interview with Tom Keighley. *Nurs Management* 6(5): 15–19

Byrt R (1994) *Consumer Participation in a Voluntary Organisation for Mental Health.* Unpublished PhD thesis, Loughborough University

Byrt R (1999) Nursing. The importance of the psychosocial environment. In: Campling P, Haigh R (eds) *Therapeutic Communities: Past, Present and Future*. Jessica Kingsley, London

Cameron A (1999) The role of interest groups. In: Masterson A, Maslin-Prothero S (eds) *Nursing and Politics. Power through Practice*. Churchill Livingstone, Edinburgh

Cameron S (1998) Whose reality is it anyway? In: Barker PJ, Davidson B (eds) *Psychiatric Nursing. Ethical Strife*. Arnold, London

Campbell-Clark A, MacIver-Campbell C, Turnbull A, Urquhart A (1923) *Handbook for Mental Nurses:(Handbook for Attendants on the Insane)*. 7th edn. Baillière, Tindall and Cox, London

Campling P (1999) Chaotic personalities. Maintaining the therapeutic alliance. In: Campling P, Haigh R (eds) *Therapeutic Communities: Past, Present and Future*. Jessica Kingsley, London

Campling P, Davies S (1997) Reflections on an English revolution. *Therapeutic Communities* **18**(1): 63–73

Campling P, Haigh R (eds) (1999) *Therapeutic Communities. Past, Present and Future*. Jessica Kingsley, London

Capewell (1992) Clinical directorates: a panacea for clinicians involved in management? *Health Bulletin* **50**(6): 441–7

Carnal CA (1990) *Managing Change in Organisations*. Prentice Hall, London

Carr W, Kemmis S (1986) *Becoming Critical – Education, Knowledge & Action Research*. The Falmer Press, UK

Castledine G (1994) Specialist and advanced nursing and the scope of practice. In: Hunt G, Wainwright P (eds) *Expanding the Role of the Nurse The Scope of Professional Practice*. Blackwell Science, Oxford

Central Nottinghamshire Healthcare NHS Trust (1999) *Newsletter For Service Users And Carers*. Central Nottinghamshire Healthcare NHS Trust, Mansfield

Cipolle RJ, Strand LM, Morley PC (1998) *Pharmaceutical Care Practice*. McGraw-Hill, New York

Dooher J, Clark A, Fowler J (eds) (2001) *Case Studies on Practice Development*. Quay Books Division, Mark Allen Publishing Ltd, Salisbury, Wiltshire

Clark VB (1999) The ABCs of highly effective presentations: a customer-centered approach. *J Nurses Staff Dev* **15**(1): 23–6

Clarke JB (1999) Evidence-based practice: a retrograde step? The importance of pluralism in evidence generation for the practice of health care. *J Clin Nurs* **8**: 89–94

Closs SJ, Cheater FM (1994) Utilisation of nursing research: culture, interest and support. *J Adv Nurs* **19**(4): 762–73

Coffey M (1997) Mental health nursing. Supervised discharge: concerns about the new powers for nurses. *Br J Nurs* **6**(4): 215–8

Coombs M, Holgate M (1998) Developing a framework for practice: a clinical perspective. In: Rolfe G, Fulbrook P (eds) *Advanced Nursing Practice.* Butterworth Heinemann, Oxford

Council of The Royal Pharmaceutical Society of Great Britain (1998) *Report of the Council.* RPSGB, London

Collins M, Robinson D (1997) Studying patient choice and privacy in a forensic setting. *Psychiatric Care* **4**(10): 12–15

Crapanzano S (1999) The advancement of nursing competence the development and implementation of nursing continuing education. *Pelican News* **55**(1): 5–6

Crapanzano S (1999) The advancement of nursing competence. *Pelican News* **55**(3): 10

Cullen E, Jones L, Woodward R (1997) *Therapeutic Communities for Offenders.* Wiley, Chichester

Cutcliffe J, Jackson A, Ward M, Cannon B, Titchen A (1998) Practice development in mental health nursing. *Mental Health Practice* **2**(4): 27–31

Day C (1993) *Research and the continuing professional development of teachers.* An inaugural lecture. University of Nottingham, School of Education

Deal T, Kennedy A (1988) *Corporate Cultures. The Rites and Rituals of Corporate Life.* Penguin Books, London. First published (1982) Addison-Wesley, USA

Denner S (1995) Extending professional practice: benefits and pitfalls. *Nurs Times* **91**(14): 27–9

Department of Health and Social Security (1980) *Report of the Review of Rampton Hospital.* Cmnd 8073 HMSO, London

Department of Health (1988) *Working Together: Securing a Quality Workforce for the NHS.* HMSO, London

Department of Health (1992a) *The Health of the Nation: A Strategy for Health in England.* HMSO, London

Department of Health (1992b) *Report of the Committee of Inquiry into Complaints About Ashworth Hospital.* HMSO, London

Department of Health and the Royal Pharmaceutical Society of Great Britain (1992) *Pharmaceutical Care: The future for community pharmacy – report of the joint working party on the future role of community pharmacy.* RPSGB, London

Department of Health (1993a) *The Challenge for Nursing and Midwifery in the 21st Century. The Heathrow Debate.* HMSO, London

Department of Health (1993b) *A Vision for the Future. The Nursing, Midwifery and Health Visiting Contribution to Health Care.* HMSO, London

Department of Health (1996) *Consultation Counts. Guidelines for Service Purchasers and Users and Carers Based on the Experience of the National User and Carer Group.* HMSO, London

Department of Health (1997) *The new NHS – modern, dependable.* HMSO, London

Department of Health (1998a) *A First Class Service; Quality in the new National Health Service.* HMSO, London

Department of Health (1998b) *Our Healthier Nation.* HMSO, London

Department of Health (1999a) *Making a Difference: Strengthening the nursing, midwifery and health visiting contribution to health & healthcare.* HMSO, London

Department of Health (1999b) *Governance in The New NHS. Controls Assurance Statements 1999/2000: Risk Management and Organisational Controls.* HMSO, London

Department of Health (1999c) *Saving Lives.* HMSO, London

Department of Health (1999d) *Health Service Circular 1999/154 Continuing Professional Development: Quality in the New NHS.* HMSO, London

Dewey J (1933) *How We Think: A Restatement of the Relation of Reflective Thinking to the Educative Process.* DC Heath, Boston

Dimond B (1990) *Legal Aspects of Nursing.* Prentice Hall International (UK) Ltd, Hemel Hempstead

Dimond B (1994) Legal aspects of role expansion. In: Hunt G, Wainwright P (eds) *Expanding the Role of the Nurse The Scope of Professional Practice.* Blackwell Science, Oxford

Dimond B (1995a) The scope of professional practice and the accident & emergency nurse. *Accid Emerg Nurs* **3**: 105–7

Dimond B (1995b) When the nurse wields the scalpel. *Br J Nurs* **4** (2): 65–6

Dimond B (1996a) *The Legal Aspects Of Child Health Care.* Mosby, London

Dimond B (1996b) *The Legal Aspects Of Midwifery.* Books For Midwives Press, London

Dimond B (1999) *Patients' Rights, Responsibilities and the Nurse.* 2nd edn. Quay Books Divison, Mark Allen Publishing Ltd, Salisbury, Wiltshire

Dimond B (2000) Legal issues arising in community nursing 4: expanded role. *Br J Com Nurs* **5**(2): 67–9

Dingwall R, Rafferty AM, Webster C, eds (1988) *An Introduction to the Social History of Nursing.* Routledge, London

Dowling S, Martin R, Skidmore P, Doyal L *et al* (1996) Nurses taking on junior doctor's work: a confusion of accountability. *Br Med J* **312**: 1211–14

Downe M (1997) Progress report. The emergence of the person in dementia research. *Ageing And Society* **17**: 597–607

Dyson L (1997) Advanced nursing roles: their worth in nursing. *Prof Nurse* **12**(10): 728–32

English National Board for Nursing, Midwifery and Health Visiting (1991) *Framework for Continuing Professional Education for Nurses, Midwives and Health Visitors.* ENB, London

English National Board for Nursing, Midwifery and Health Visiting (1993a) *Report of the Taskforce: Strategy for Research.* ENB, London

English National Board for Nursing, Midwifery and Health Visiting (1993b) *The Board's Response to the Strategy for Research.* ENB, London

Ericsson K, Smith J (1991) *Toward a General Theory of Expertise.* Cambridge University Press, Cambridge

Estabrooks CA (1998) Will evidence-based nursing practice make practice perfect? *Can J Nurs Res* **30**(1): 15–36

Fatchett A (1998) *Nursing In The New NHS.* Ballière Tindall, Edinburgh

Festinger L (1957) *A Theory of Cognitive Dissonance.* Harper and Row, New York

Försterling F (1995) Control In: Manstead ASR, Hewstone M (eds) *The Blackwell Encyclopaedia Of Social Psychology.* Blackwells, Oxford

Fowler J (1996) Clinical supervision: What do you do after you say hello? *Br J Nurs* **5**(6): 382–5

Fowler J (1998) *The Handbook of Clinical Supervision – Your questions answered.* Quay Books Division, Mark Allen Publishing Ltd, Salisbury,Wiltshire

Fowler J, Chevannes M (1998) Evaluating the efficacy of reflective practice within the context of clinical supervision. *J Adv Nurs* **27**(2): 379–82

Fraher A, Limpinnian M (1999) User empowerment within mental health nursing. In: Wilkinson G, Miers M (eds) *Power and Nursing Practice.* Macmillian, Basingstoke

Freshwater D (1998) *Transformatory Learning in Nurse Education.* Unpublished PhD Thesis, University of Nottingham

Furze G, Pearcey P (1999) Continuing education in nursing: a review of the literature. *J Adv Nurs* **29**(2): 355–63

Garbett R (1998) Do the right thing. *Nurs Times* **94**(27): 828–29

Gascoine v Ian Sheridan and Co (a firm) and Latham (QBD: Mitchell J) [1995] 5 Med LR 437. In: Tingle J (1997b) Legal problems in the operating theatre: learning from mistakes. *Br J Nurs* **6**(15): 889–91

General Medical Council (1995) *Duties of a Doctor, Good Medical Practice* (clause 28). GMC, London

Gibson CH (1995) The process of empowerment in mothers of chronically ill children. *J Adv Nurs* **21**: 1201–10

Giles PF, Moran V (1989) Preceptor program evaluation demonstrates improved orientation. *J Nurs Staff Dev* **5**(1): 17–24

Glover D (1998) The art of practice development. *Nurs Times* **94**(36): 58–9

Godfrey J (1999) Empowerment through sexuality. In: Wilkinson G, Miers M (eds) *Power and Nursing Practice*. Macmillian, Basingstoke

Godin P, Scanlon C (1997) Supervision and control: a community psychiatric nursing perspective. *J Mental Health* **6**(1): 75–84

Godsell M (1999) Caring for people with learning disabilities. In: Wilkinson G, Miers M (eds) *Power and Nursing Practice*. Macmillian, Basingstoke

Goffman E (1968) *Asylums. Essays On The Social Situation Of Mental Patients And Others.* Penguin Books, Harmondsworth

Goodman D (1997) Application of the critical pathway and integrated case teaching method to nursing orientation. *J Cont Educ Nurs* **28**(5): 205–10

Goodyer L, Lovejoy A, Nathan A, Warnett S (1996) Medicines management: 'Brown bag' medication reviews in community pharmacies. *Pharma J* **256**: 723–5

Gould D, Chamberlain A (1997) The use of a ward-based educational teaching package to enhance nurses' compliance with infection control procedures. *J Clin Nurs* **6**(1): 55–67

Gordon M (1998) Empowerment and breastfeeding. In: Kendall S (ed) *Health and Empowerment. Research and Practice.* Arnold, London

Gostin L (1985) Introduction: a policy overview. In: Gostin L (ed) *Secure Provision. A Review of Special Services for the Mentally Ill and Mentally Handicapped in England and Wales.* Tavistock, London

Gramling L, Nugent K (1998) Teaching caring within the context of health. *Nurse Educator* **23**(2): 47–51

Gray J (1997) *Evidence-Based Healthcare.* Churchill Livingstone, Edinburgh

Grealish M, O'Down T (1998) General practitioners and women with urinary incontinence. *Br J Gen Prac* **48**: 975–8

Green J, Coupland B, Kitzinger J (1998) *Great Expectations: A Prospective Study of Women's Expectations and Experiences of Childbirth.* Child Care and Development Group, Cambridge

Greenhalgh T, Douglas H-R (1999) Experiences of general practitioners and practice nurses of training courses in evidence based health care: a qualitative study. *Br J Gen Prac* **49**: 536–40

Greenwood J (1998) The role of reflection in single and double loop learning. *J Adv Nurs* **27**: 1048–53

Gross RD (1988) *Psychology: The Science of Mind and Behaviour.* Arnold, London

Gunn J, Taylor PJ (eds) (1995) *Forensic Psychiatry. Clinical, Legal And Ethical Issues.* Butterworth-Heinemann, Oxford

Hall SM, Holloway IM (1998) Staying in control: women's experiences of labour in water. *Midwifery* **14**(1): 30–6

Hampden-Turner C (1990) *Corporate Culture – From Vicious to Virtuous Circles.* The Economist Books Ltd, London

Handy C (1993) *Understanding Organisations.* 4th edn. Penguin Books, Harmondsworth

Hanily F (1995) A new approach to practice development in mental health. *Nurs Times* **91**(21): 34–5

Harvey J (1991) An evaluation of approaches to assess the quality of nursing care using (predetermined) quality assurance tools. *J Adv Nurs* **16**(3): 277–86

Haworth S (1998) Practice leaders. *Nurs Manag* **4**(8): 25

Helgerson S (1992) Feminine principles of leadership: The perfect fit for nursing revolution. *J Nurse Empowerment* **2**(2): 50–135

Helman C (1994) *Culture Health and Illness.* 3rd edn. Butterworth-Heinemann, Oxford

Henry JM (1997) Gaming: a teaching strategy to enhance adult learning. *J Cont Educ Nurs* **28**(5): 231–4

Hepler CD, Strand LM (1990) Opportunities and responsibilities in pharmaceutical care. *Am J Hosp Pharm* **47**: 533–43

Hepler CD (1992) The future of pharmacy: Pharmaceutical care (Appendix). In: Smith MC, Knapp DA (eds) *Pharmacy, Drugs and Medical Care.* Williams and Wilkins, Baltimore

Heron J (1998) *Sacred Science.* PCCS Books, Ross on Wye

Heron J (1990) *Helping the Client. A Creative Practical Guide.* SAGE Publications, London

Hinshelwood RD (1999) Psychoanalytic origins and today's work: the cassel heritage. In: Campling P, Haigh R (eds) *Therapeutic Communities. Past, Present and Future.* Jessica Kingsley, London

Hodnett ED (1998) *Continuity of caregivers during pregnancy & childbirth* (Cochrane review). In: The Cochrane Library, Issue 4. Update Software, Oxford

Hofstede J (1991) *Cultures and Organisations: Software of the mind – Intercultural co-operation and its importance for survival.* Saga, Beverley Hills, California

Hovland CI, Janis IL, Kelly HH (1953) *Communication and Persuasion.* Yale University Press, New Haven, CT

Hunt J (1981) Indicators for nursing practice: the use of research findings. *J Adv Nurs* **6**(3): 189–94

Hunt S, Symonds A (1995) *The Social Meaning of Midwifery.* MacMillan, Basingstoke

Hunt G (1995) *Whistleblowing in The Health Service. Accountability, Law and Professional Practice.* Edward Arnold, London

Iqbal Z, Clarke M, Taylor D (1998) Clinical effectiveness: the potential for change in maternity care. *J Clin Effect* **3**(2): 67–71

Jackson A, Ward M, Cutcliffe J, Titchen A *et al* (1999a) Practice development in mental health nursing: part two. *Mental Health Practice* **2**(5): 20–5

Jackson A, Cutcliffe J, Ward M, Titchen A *et al* (1999b) Practice development in mental health nursing: part three. *Mental Health Practice* **2**(7): 24–5

Jarvis P, Gibson S (1997) *The Teacher Practitioner and Mentor in Nursing, Midwifery, Health Visiting and the Social Services.* 2nd edn. Stanley Thornes, Cheltenham

Jary D, Jary J (1995) *Collins Dictionary Of Sociology.* 2nd edn. Harper Collins, Glasgow

Jenkinson C (1997) *Assessment and Evaluation of Health and Medical Care.* Open University Press, Buckingham

Johns C (1998) Opening the doors of perception. In: Johns C, Freshwater D (eds) *Transforming Nursing through Reflective Practice.* Blackwell Scientific, Oxford

Johns C, Freshwater D (eds) (1998) *Transforming Nursing through Reflective Practice.* Blackwell Scientific, Oxford

Johns C (1995) The value of reflective practice in nursing. *J Clin Nurs* **4**: 23–30

Johnson J, Scholes K (1993) *Exploring Corporate Strategy.* 3rd edn. Prentice Hall, London

Johnson M (1999) Racism and reform. *NursTimes* **95**(19): 25

Jones IF (1 998) Community pharmacy and the National Health Service. *Pharma J Suppl* NHS24-NHS27

Jones K (1993) *Asylums And After. A Revised History of the Mental Health Services from the Early Eighteenth Century to the Nineteen Nineties.* The Athlone Press, London

Kelham I (1999) Incontinence: potential of practice nurses. *Prac Nurs* **10**(1): 33–4

Kendall S, ed (1998a) *Health And Empowerment. Research And Practice.* Arnold, London

Kendall S (1998b) Introduction. In: Kendall S (ed) *Health And Empowerment. Research And Practice.* Arnold, London

Kettle C, Johanson R (1999) Absorbable synthetic versus catgut suture material for perineal repair (Cochrane Review) In: The Cochrane Library, Issue 2, Update Software, Oxford

Keyzer D, Wright S (1998) Change strategies: the classic models. In: Wright SG (ed) *Changing Nursing Practice*. 2nd edn. Arnold, London

Kirkham M (1989) Midwives and information-giving during labour. In: Robinson S, Thompson A (eds) *Midwives, Research & Childbirth: vol. 1*. Chapman and Hall, London

Kirkham M (1995) Using personal planning to meet the challenge of changing childbirth. In: *The Challenge of Changing Childbirth: midwifery educational resource pack*. Section 1. ENB, London

Kitson A, Currie L (1996) Clinical practice development and research activities in four health authorities. *J Clin Nurs* **5**: 41–51

Kitwood T (1997) *Dementia Reconsidered*. Open University Press, Milton Keynes

Kitson A, Ahmed LA, Harvey G, Seers K *et al* (1996) From research to practice: One organisational method for promoting research-based practice. *J Adv Nurs* **23**: 430–40

Kitson A, Harvey G, McCormack B (1998) Enabling the implementation of evidence-based practice: a conceptual framework. *Quality in Health Care* **7**(3): 149–58

Kohner N (1994) *Clinical Supervision in Practice*. King's Fund Centre, London

Knight R, Procter S (1999) Implementation of clinical guidelines for female urinary incontinence: a comparative analysis of organisational structures and service delivery. *Health & Social Care* **7**(4): 280–90

Lancaster J, Lancaster W (eds) (1982) *The Nurse as a Change Agent*. CV Mosby, St Louis

Land L, Mhaolrunaigh MA, Castledine G (1996) Extent and effectiveness of the scope of professional practice. *Nurs Times* **92**(35): 32–5

Largo-Janssen T, Smits A, van Weel C (1990) Women with urinary incontinence: self perceived worries and GPs knowledge of problems. *Br J Gen Prac* **40**: 331–4

Latter S (1998) Health promotion in the acute setting: the case for empowering nurses. In: Kendall S (ed) (1998a) *Health and Empowerment. Research and Practice*. Arnold, London

Leiba T (1998) The effects of mental health legislation, 1890–1990. *Int Hist Nurs J* **3**(4): 12–18

Leicestershire and Rutland Healthcare NHS Trust (1999) *Information Booklet. Internal Document. Leicester*. Leicestershire and Rutland Healthcare NHS Trust, Leicester

Lewis J, Glennerster H (1996) *Implementing The New Community Care*. Open University Press, Milton Keynes

Littlewood R, Lipsedge M (1997) *Aliens and Alienists*. 3rd edn. Routledge, London

Lowe T (1992) Characteristics of effective nursing interventions in the management of challenging behaviour. *J Adv Nurs* **17**: 1226–32

Luker K (ed) (1992) *Health Visiting: Towards community health nursing*. 2nd edn. Blackwells, Oxford

Lumby J (1998) Transforming nursing through reflective practice. In: Johns C, Freshwater D (eds) *Transforming Nursing Through Reflective Practice*. Blackwell Science, Oxford

Lunn J (1994) The scope of professional practice from a legal perspective. *Br J Nurs* **3**(15): 770–2

McCann G (1998) Control in the community. In: Mason T, Mercer D (eds) *Critical Perspectives in Forensic Care. Inside Out*. Macmillian, Basingstoke

Mackie C (1999) Milliennium career options for pharmacists. *Pharma J* **262**: 119–21

Magennis C, Slevin E, Cunningham J (1999) Nurses' attitudes to the extension and expansion of their clinical roles. *Nurs Standard* **13**(51): 32–6

Maguire T (1995) Broad spectrum: Pharmaceutical care – who pays? *Pharma J* **254**: 642

Manning NP (1989) *The Therapeutic Community Movement: Charisma and Routinisation*. Routledge, London

Marks S (1997) The legacy of the history of nursing for post-apartheid South Africa. In: Rafferty AM, Robinson J, Elkan R (eds) *Nursing History and The Politics of Welfare*. Routledge, London

Marquis BL, Huston CJ (1996) *Leadership Roles and Management Functions in Nursing*. 2nd edn. Lippincott, Philadelphia

Martin JP (1984) *Hospitals In Trouble*. Blackwell, Oxford

Mason T, Chandley M (1990) Nursing models in a special hospital: a critical study of efficacity. *J Adv Nurs* **15**: 667–73

Mason T (1997) An ethnomethodological analysis of the use of seclusion. *J Adv Nurs* **26**: 780–9

Mason T, Mercer D (eds) (1998) *Critical Perspectives In Forensic Care. Inside Out*. Macmillan, Basingstoke

Mason T, Chandley M (1999) *Managing Violence And Aggression. A Manual for Nurses and Health Care Workers*. Churchill Livingstone, Edinburgh

Mason P (1999) Pharmaceutical care in Minnesota – a profoundly different experience. *Pharma J* **262**: 705–8

Maslin-Prothero S, Masterson A (1999) Power, politics and nursing. In: Masterson A, Maslin-Prothero S (eds) *Nursing and Politics. Power through Practice.* Churchill-Livingstone, Edinburgh

McElnay J (1998) Getting pharmaceutical care into community practice. *Pharma J* **261**: 570

McFadyen J, Farrington A (1997) User and carer participation in the NHS. *Br J Health Care Man* **3**(5): 260–4

McGregor-Kettles A, Russell JH (1996) User views of a forensic service. *Psychiatr Care* **3**(3): 98–104

McHugh A, Wain I, West M (1995) Handle with care. *Nurs Times* **91**(6): 62–3

McLeod J (1996) The humanistic paradigm. In: Woolfe R, Dryden W (eds) *Handbook of Counselling Psychology.* Sage, London

Mercer D (1998) Beyond madness and badness: where angels fear to tread? In: Mason T, Mercer D (eds) *Critical Perspectives In Forensic Care. Inside Out.* Macmillan, Basingstoke

Miles A, Bentley P, Price N, Polychronis A *et al* (1996) Methods of auditing the totality of patient care 1: pre-requisite management structures and organisational innovations. In: Miles A, Lugon M (eds) (1996) *Effective Clinical Practice.* Blackwell, Oxford

Monkman J, Hempstead N (1999) Throw light on two new government papers. *Nurs Management* **6**(6): 6

Moores Y (1999) New look for 21st century nurse. *Nurs Times* **95**(28): 5

Morgan P, Potter C (1995) Professional cultures & paradigms of quality in health care. In: Kirkpatrick I, Martinez M (eds) *The Politics of Quality in Health Care.* Routledge, London

Morris P (1969) *Put Away. A Sociological Study of Institutions for the Mentally Retarded.* Routledge and Kegan Paul, London

Morrison P (1996) Issues for clinical leaders in nursing development units. *Nurs Times* **92**(12): 37–9

Morrison P, Burnard P, Philips C (1996) Patient satisfaction in a forensic unit. *J Mental Health* **5**(4): 369–77

Mulhall A (1995) Nursing research: what difference does it make? *J Adv Nurs* **21**(3): 576–83

Munro R (2000) Going through the roof. *Nurs Times* **96**(4): 10

National Health Service Executive (1996) *Promoting Clinical Effectiveness: A Framework for Action in and Throughout the NHS.* Department of Health, London

National Health Service Executive (1998a) *Better Health and Better Health Care: Implementing the new NHS and Our Healthier Nation.* HSC 1998/021. February 25 1998. Health Service Circular. Department of Health, London

National Health Service Executive (1998b) *A Consultation on a Strategy for Nursing, Midwifery and Health Visiting.* HSC 1998/045, April 20 1998 Health Service Circular, Department of Health, London

National Health Service Executive (1998c) *Integrating Theory and Practice in Nursing.* NHS Executive, London

National Health Service Executive (1998d) *Achieving Effective Practice: A Clinical Effectiveness and Research Information Pack.* Department of Health, London

National Practice Development Network (1999) *Development and Evaluative Approaches to Mental Health in Acute In-Patient Care.* King's College, London.

Nolan P (1995) Mental health nursing-origins and developments. In: Baly M (ed) *Nursing and Social Change.* Routledge, London

Nolan M, Grant G (1993) Action research and quality of care: a mechanism for agreeing basic values as a precursor to change. *J Adv Nurs* **18**: 305–11

North C, Ritchie J, Ward K (1993) *Factors influencing the implementation of the care programme approach.* HMSO, London

Norton K, Hinshelwood RD (1996) Severe personality disorder: treatment issues and selection for inpatient psychotherapy. *Br J Psych* **168**: 723–31

Norton PA, MacDonald LD, Sedgwick PM, Stanton SL (1998) Distress and delay associated with urinary incontinence, frequency and urgency in women. *Br Med J* **297**: 1187–9

Nursing Times (1999) Comment. *Nurs Times* **95**(28): 3

Oakley A (1993) *Essays on Women, Medicine and Health.* Edinburgh University Press, Edinburgh

O'Brien J, Austin M, Sethi P, O'Boyle P (1991) Urinary incontinence: prevalence, need for treatment and effectiveness of intervention by nurses. *Br Med J* **303**: 1308–12

Odibo L (1997) Suturing of perineal trauma: how well are we doing – an audit. *Br J Midwifery* **5**(11): 690–2

Osbourne P (1996) Research in nursing education. In: Cormack DFS (1996) (ed) *The Research Process in Nursing.* Blackwell Scientific, Oxford

Ostell A, Oakland S (1999) Absolutist thinking and health. *Br J Med Psychol* **72**: 239–50

Ourousoff A (1992) In article: Prisoners of corporate culture by Roger Trapp. *Independent on Sunday*, 2nd August

Øvretveit J (1997) How patient power and client participation affects relations between practitioners. In: Øvretveit J, Mathias P, Thompson T (eds) *Interprofessional Working for Health and Social Care.* Macmillan, Basingstoke

Oxman A (1995) No magic bullets. *Can Med Assoc J* **153**: 1423–31

Page S (1995) Practice development units: progress update. *Nurs Standard* **10**(3): 25–28

Parahoo K (1999) Research Utilisation and attitudes towards research among psychiatric nurses in Northern Ireland. *J Psych Mental Health Nurs* **6**: 125–35

Payne R, Couzens I (1987) *Stress in Health Professionals*. Wiley, New York

Peach L (chair) (1993) *Fitness for Practice: The UKCC Commission for Nursing and Midwifery Education*. United Kingdom Central Council for Nursing, Midwifery and Health Visiting, London

Pearson A (1995) A history of nursing development units. In: Salvage J, Wright SG (eds) *Nursing Development Units. A Force for Change*. Scutari Press, London

Pearson A (1997) An evaluation of the King's Fund centre nursing development unit network 1989–91. *J Clin Nurs* **6**: 25–33

Pearson GA (1987) Business ethics: implications for continuing education/ staff development practice. *J Cont Educ Nurs* **18**(1): 20–4

Peckham M (1991) Research and Development for the National Health Service. *Lancet* **338**: 367–71

Pedler M, Burgoyne J, Boydell T (1986) *A Manager's Guide To Self-Development*. 2nd edn. McGraw-Hill Book Company Ltd, Berkshire

Peters TJ, Waterman JHR (1982) *In Search of Excellence. Lessons from America's Best-Run Companies*. Harper Row: New York

Peters T (1993) *Liberation Management*. Pan, London

Pharmaceutical Services Negotiating Committee (1998) *Developing Patient Care: Medicine Management in Community Pharmacy – Report of the Working Party*. PSNC, Aylesbury

Philp M (1996) Power. In: Kuper A, Kuper J (eds) *The Social Science Encyclopaedia*. 2nd edn. Routledge, London

Phillips R, Donald A, Mousseau-Gershman Y, Powell T (1998) Applying theory to practice – the use of 'ripple effect' plans in continuing education. *Nur Educ Today* **18**(1): 12–9

Pilgrim D (1995) Explaining abuse and inadequate care. In: Hunt G (ed) *Whistleblowing in the Health Service. Accountability, Law and Professional Practice*. Arnold, London

Polit D, Hungler B (1995) *Nursing Research – Principles and Methods*. Lippincott, Philadelphia

Power KJ (1997) The legal and ethical implications of consent to nursing procedures. *Br J Nurs* **6**(15): 885–8

Pratt KJ, Bennett SG (1990) *Elements of Personnel Management*. Chapman and Hall, London

Proctor B (1986) Supervision: a cooperative exercise in accountability. In: Marken M, Payne M (eds) *Enabling and Ensuring*. Leicester National Youth Bureau and Council for Education and Training in Youth and Community Work, Leicester

Pringle J (1980) Breaking an old taboo. Guest Column. *The Times*, 26 June

Radley AS, Hall J (1994) The establishment and evaluation of a pharmacist-developed anticoagulant clinic. *Pharma J* **252**: 91–2

Redfern S, Stevens W (1998) Nursing development units: their structure and orientation. *J Clin Nurs* **7**: 218–26

Rafferty AM (1996) *The Politics Of Nursing Knowledge*. Routledge, London

Re F [1990] 2 AC 1 In: Dowling S, Martin R, Skidmore P, Doyal L *et al* (1996) Nurses taking on junior doctor's work: a confusion of accountability. *Br Med J* **312**: 1211–14

Robb B (1967) *Sans Everything. A Case to Answer*. Nelson, London

Robinson J (1993) *The Individual And Society. A Marxist Approach to Human Psychology*. Index Academic, London

Roe B, Webb C (eds) (1998) *Research and Development in Clinical Nursing Practice*. Whurr, London

Rogers E (1983, 1995) *The Diffusion of Innovations*. The Free Press, New York

Rolfe G (1996) *Closing the Theory-Practice Gap. A New Paradigm for Nursing*. Butterworth Heinemann, Oxford

Rolfe G (1998a) Advanced practice and the reflective nurse: developing knowledge out of practice. In: Rolfe G, Fulbrook P (eds) *Advanced Nursing Practice*. Butterworth Heinemann, Oxford

Rolfe G (1998b) *Expanding Nursing Knowledge*. Butterworth Heinemann, Oxford

Rolfe G (1998c) The theory-practice gap in nursing: from research-based practice to practitioner-based research. *J Adv Nurs* **28**(3): 672–9

Royal College of Nursing (1996) *Clinical Effectiveness: A Royal College of Nursing Guide*. RCN, London

Royal College of Nursing (1997) *The Cost of Continence*. RCN, London

Royal Pharmaceutical Society of Great Britain and Merck Sharp & Dohme (1997) *From Compliance to Concordance: Achieving Shared Goals in Medicine Taking – Report of the Working Party*. RPSGB, London

Royal Pharmaceutical Society of Great Britain (1995) *Pharmacy in a New Age: Developing a Strategy for the Future of Pharmacy*. RPSGB, London

Royal Pharmaceutical Society of Great Britain (1996) *Pharmacy in a New Age: The New Horizon*. RPSGB, London

Royal Pharmaceutical Society of Great Britain (1997) *Pharmacy in a New Age: Building the Future*. RPSGB, London

Royal Pharmaceutical Society of Great Britain (1999) *Medicines, Ethics and Practice: A Guide for Pharmacists.* 21st edn. RPSGB, London

Royal Pharmaceutical Society of Great Britain (1999) Models of remuneration for pharmaceutical services in the community. *Pharma J* **262**: 75–9

Russell JH, McGregor-Kettles A (1996) User views of a forensic service. *Psych Care* **3**(3): 98–104

Ryles S (1999) A concept analysis of empowerment. *J Adv Nurs* **29**(3): 600–7

Salvage J, Wright SG (1995) *Nursing Development Units. A Force for Change.* Scutari Press, London

Sayce L (1995) Response to violence: a framework for fair treatment. In: Crichton J (ed) *Psychiatric Patient Violence. Risk And Response.* Duckworth, London

Scambler G (ed) (1997) *Sociology as Applied to Medicine.* WB Saunders, London

Scott G (1999) *Change Matters: making a difference in education and training.* Allen and Unwin, St Leonards, NSW

Seim A, Sivertsen B, Eriksen B, Hunskaar S (1996) Treatment of urinary incontinence in women in general practice: observational study. *Br Med J* **312**: 1459–62

Senior B (1997) *Organisational Change.* Pitman Publishing, London

Sermer R, Raines D (1997) Positioning during the second stage of labour: Moving back to basics. *J Obstet Gynaecol Neonatal Nurs* **26**(6): 727–34

Scholes J (1996) Staff Role Transition and Emotional Labour in NDUs. *Nurs Times* **92**(31): 40–3

Schön DA (1983) *The Reflective Practitioner.* Temple Smith, London

Schön DA (1987) *Educating the Reflective Practitioner.* Jossey Bass, San Francisco

Shepperd S, Doll H, Jenkinson C (1997) Randomized controlled trials. In: Scott C (1999) A description of the roles, activities and skills of clinical nurse specialists in the united states. *Clin Nur Special* **13**(4): 183–90

Shepherd T (1999) Management opportunities. *Nurs Management* **6**(6): 5

Shirley KE, Mander R (1996) The power of language. *Br J Midwifery* **4**(5): 298–300, 317–18

Shuldham C (1997) The leadership challenge in nursing. *Nurs Management* **3**(10): 14–7

Simpson D (1997) Pharmaceutical care: the Minnesota model. *Pharma J* **258**: 899–904

Skultans V (1998) Anthropology and Narrative. In: Greenhalgh T, Hurwitz B (eds) *Narrative Based Medicine.* BMA, London

Slevin E, Sines D (1996) Attitudes of nurses in a general hospital towards people with learning disabilities. *J Adv Nurs* **24**: 1116–26.

Small JA, Geldart K, Gutman G, Clarke Scott MA (1998) The discourse of self in dementia. *Ageing and Society* **18**: 291–316

Smith PB (1995) Social influence processes. In: Argyle M, Colman AM (eds) *Social Psychology*. Longman, London

Smith MC, Knapp DA (1992) *Pharmacy, Drugs and Medical Care*. Williams and Wilkins, Baltimore

Smith P (ed) (1997) *Research Mindedness for Practice: An interactive approach for nursing and health care*. Churchill Livingstone, London

Smith P (ed) (1998) *Nursing Research: Setting New Agendas*. Edward Arnold, London

Sparrow S, Robinson J (1992) The use and limitations of Phaneuf's Nursing Audit. *J Adv Nurs* **17**(12): 1479–88

Stephen H (1999) Consultants medical and nursing. *Nurs Standard* **13**(28): 12–3

Stern G (1992) Invisible horse – are they limiting your growth? *J Nurs Empowerment* **2**(2): 86–91

Stitt P (1995) Development Of the lecturer/practitioner role. In: Kendrick, K, Weir P, Rosser E (eds) *Innovations in Nursing Practice*. Edward Arnold, London

Strickland OL, Fishman DJ (1994) *Nursing Issues in the 1990s*. Delmar, New York

Sullivan P (1997) Mental health nursing. The care programme approach: a nursing perspective. *Br J Nurs* **6**(4): 208, 210–4

Sullivan P (1998) Developing evidence-based care in mental health nursing. *Nurs Standard* **12**(31): 35–8

Symonds B (1998) The philosophical and social context of mental health care and legislation. *J Adv Nurs* **27**:945–54

Tann J, Blenkinsopp A, Allen J, Platt, A (1996) Leading edge practitioners in community pharmacy: Approaches to innovation. *Int J Pharm Prac* **4**: 235–45

Tennant A, Hughes G (1998) Men talking about dysfunctional masculinity: an innovative approach to working with aggressive personality disordered offender-patients. *Psych Care* **5**(3): 92–9

Thacker S, Stroup D, Peterson H (1999) *Continuous electronic fetal heart monitoring during labour* (Cochrane review). In: The Cochrane Library, Issue 2, Update Software, Oxford

Tingle J (1997a) Expanded role of the nurse: accountability confusion. *Br J Nurs* **6**(17): 1011–3

Tingle J (1997b) Legal problems in the operating theatre: learning from mistakes. *Br J Nurs* **6**(15): 889 –91

Thomas T, Plyman K *et al* (1988) Prevalence of urinary incontinence *Br Med J* **281**: 243–5

Thompson A (1995) Maternal behaviour during spontaneous and directed pushing in the second stage of labour. *J Adv Nurs* **22**: 1027–34

Thompson P (1972) *Bound For Broadmoor.* Hodder and Stoughton, London

Thomson M, Oxman A *et al* (1998) *Audit and feedback to improve health professional practice and health care outcomes* (Part 2). In: The Cochrane Library, Issue 3, Update Software, Oxford

Thomson A (1996) Editorial. A fight for childbearing women to be treated with dignity and respect. *Midwifery* **12**(1): 6

Todd G, Freshwater D (1999) Reflective practice and guided discovery: models for clinical supervision. *Br J Nurs* **8**(2): 1383–89

Tones K (1998) Empowerment for health. The challenge. In: Kendall S (ed) *Health and Empowerment. Research and Practice.* Edward Arnold, London

Tones K, Tilford S (1994) *Health Education. Effectiveness, Efficiency and Equity.* 2nd edn. Chapman and Hall, London

United Kingdom Central Council for Nursing, Midwifery and Health Visiting (1989) *Exercising Accountability.* UKCC, London

United Kingdom Central Council for Nursing, Midwifery and Health Visiting (1992a) *Code of Professional Conduct.* UKCC, London

United Kingdom Central Council for Nursing, Midwifery and Health Visiting (1992b) *The Scope of Professional Practice.* UKCC, London

United Kingdom Central Council for Nursing, Midwifery and Health Visiting (1995a) *Standards for Post-registration Education and Practice.* UKCC, London

United Kingdom Central Council for Nursing, Midwifery and Health Visiting (1995b) *PREP & YOU Fact Sheet 3.* UKCC, London

United Kingdom Central Council for Nursing, Midwifery and Health Visiting (1996a) *Position Statement on Clinical Supervision for Nursing and Health Visiting.* UKCC, London

United Kingdom Central Council for Nursing, Midwifery and Health Visiting (1996b) *Guidelines For Professional Practice.* UKCC, London

United Kingdom Central Council for Nursing, Midwifery and Health Visiting (1998) *Midwives Rules and Code of Practice.* UKCC, London

United Kingdom Central Council for Nursing, Midwifery and Health Visiting (1999a) *The Continuing Professional Development Standard: Information for Registered Nurses, Midwives and Health Visitors.* UKCC, London

United Kingdom Central Council for Nursing, Midwifery and Health Visiting (1999b) *Fitness for Practice.* UKCC, London van Manen M (1977) *Linking Ways of Knowing with Ways of Being Practical.* State University of New York Press, New York

VÄLimÄki M, Suominen T, Peate I (1998) Attitudes of professionals, students and the general public to HIV/AIDS and people with HIV/AIDS: a review of the research. *J Adv Nurs* **27**(4): 752–9

Verma GK, Beard RM (1981) *What is Educational Research? Perspectives Techniques of Research.* Gower, Aldershot

Wahl OF (1995) *Media Madness. Public Images of Mental Illness.* Rutgers University Press, New Brunswick, New Jersey

Walsh D (ed) (1997) *Handbook of Evidence-Based Guidelines for Midwife-Led Care in Labour.* LRI NHS Trust, Leicester

Walsh M, Walsh A (1998) Practice development units: a study of team-work. *Nurs Stand* **12**(33): 35–8

Walsh, M, Ford P (1989) *Nursing Rituals, Research and Rational Actions.* Butterworth Heinemann, Oxford

Walsh M, Walsh A (1998) Practice development units: a study of teamwork. *Nurs Standard* **12**(33): 35–8

Ward M (1995) *The Leicester Project – Internal Report.* RCN Institute, Oxford

Ward M, Titchen A, Morell C, McCormack B, Kitson A (1998) Using a supervisory framework to support and evaluate a multi-project practice development programme. *J Clin Nurs* **7**: 29–36

Waterman H, Webb C, Williams A (1995) Changing nursing and nursing change: a dialectical analysis of an action research project, educational action research. In: Wells JSG (1998) Severe mental illness, statutory supervision and mental health nursing in the United Kingdom. *J Adv Nurs* **27**: 698–706

White T (1993) *Management for Clinicians.* Edward Arnold, Kent

White K, Eagle J, McNeil H, Dance S *et al* (1998) What are the factors that influence learning in relation to nursing practice? *J Nurses in Staff Dev* **14**(3): 147–53

Whittington R, Balsamo D (1998) Violence: fear and power. In: Mason T, Mercer D (eds) *Critical Perspectives in Forensic Care. Inside Out.* Macmillian, Basingstoke

Wicks S (1998) *Nurses And Doctors at Work. Rethinking Professional Boundaries.* Open University Press, Buckingham

Wilkinson G (1999) Theories of power. In: Wilkinson G, Miers M (eds) *Power and Nursing Practice.* Macmillian, Basingstoke

Wilkinson G, Miers M (eds) (1999a) *Power and Nursing Practice.* Macmillan, Basingstoke

Wilkinson G, Miers M (1999b) Power and professions. In: Wilkinson G, Miers M (eds) *Power and Nursing Practice.* Macmillan, Basingstoke

Wilsher v Essex Area Health Authority [1988] HL 1 All ER 871. In: Dimond B (1995a) The scope of professional practice and the accident & emergency nurse. *Accid Emerg Nurs* **3**: 105–7

Wilsher v Essex Area Health Authority [1986] 3 All ER 801 In: Dowling S, Martin R, Skidmore P, Doyal L *et al* (1996) Nurses taking on junior doctor's work: a confusion of accountability. *Br Med J* **312**:1211–14

Wish (1999) *Annual Report 1997–1998*. Wish, London

Wright SG (1998a) The change obstacle course: additional perspectives on the change process. In: Wright SG (ed) *Changing Nursing Practice*. 2nd edn. Edward Arnold, London

Wright SG (1998b) Nursing development units. In: Wright SG (ed) *Changing Nursing Practice*. 2nd edn. Edward Arnold, London

Wright S (1994) Nursing development units. In: Lathlean J, Vaughan B, (eds) *Unifying Nursing Practice and Theory*. Butterworth Heinemann, Oxford

Wright S (1996) The need to develop nursing practice through innovation and change. *Intern J Nurs Prac* **2**: 142–8

Yates M (1999) *Leadership Truth and Process*. www.leader-values.com

Zimbardo PG, Leippe MR (1991) *The Psychology of Attitude Change and Social Influence*. McGraw-Hill Inc, New York

Appendix

Useful addresses, contacts and sources for information

National Institute for Clinical Excellence (NICE)
11 The Strand, London WC2N 5HR
Tel 020 7766 9191
www.nice.org.uk

Promoting Action on Clinical Effectiveness (PACE)
Kings Fund, 11–13 Cavendish Square, London, W1M 0AN
Tel 020 7307 2400
email: hhutton@kefh.org.uk

NHS Centre for Reviews and Dissemination
www.york.ac.uk/inst/crd
email: revdis@york.ac.uk

Netting the Evidence
www.shef.ac.uk/sharr/ir/netting

Electronic databases

Medline
Cumulative Index of Nursing and Allied Healthcare Literature CINAHL

Internet sites

www.man.ac.uk/rcn
The Royal College of Nursing Research and Development Co-ordinating Centre
www.herts.ac.uk/lis/subjects/health/ebm.htm

Evidence-based medicine databases:

www.cochrane.co.uk
The 'Gold standard' international collaboration to establish and record good practice in evidence-based health

www.enb.org.uk
Contains the ENB's healthcare database, of particular interest to nurses.

www.infopoems.com
The 'POEM' database ('Patient Orientated Evidence that Matters')

www.ncbi.nlm.nih.gov/pubmed
way of accessing the full power of the Medline database

www.bmj.com
As well as the British Medical Journal, this gives access to evidence-based reviews such as Bandolier

www.hsrc.org.uk
Information about NICE, Clinical Governance, National Service Frameworks etc.

Index

peer review 62
personal development 29
personal development plan 67–68
personal practice 66
pharmaceutical care practice 130
pharmacy culture 123
pharmacy practice 127
political agenda 100, 126
political framework 100
Position Statement On Clinical
  Supervision For Nursing And
  Health Visiting (UKCC, 1996)
  156
Post Registration Education and
  Practice (PREP) 5
postgraduate education 127
power 4, 29, 70, 72–74, 84, 111,
  190
  ~ institutional and community
  85
practice 4, 33, 54, 79, 97, 124,
  133–135, 139, 164, 169, 170,
  177, 179, 181, 185, 192
  ~ advanced 38
  ~ best 91
  ~ changes in 130, 176
  ~ community 126
  ~ development and
    improvement 77
  ~ development of 35
  ~ innovative 13
  ~ placement experience 114
practice audit 180
practice-based pharmacists 121,
  127
practice developers 145–147, 150,
  151
practice development ix, xv, 3,
  5–6, 18, 24, 31, 69, 73, 86, 89,

91, 95, 132–133, 136, 138, 140,
  141, 145, 1 93
  ~ hospital-based 28
  ~ multi-disciplinary 100
  ~ perception of 49
practice development nurse ix, xvi,
  8, 9, 10, 28, 156
  ~ as catalyst 15
  ~ essential skills 11
  ~ skills and attributes 15
practice development unit (PDU)
  105–107, 112, 113, 114,
  116–118, 187
  ~ accreditation 116
  ~ structure 110
  ~ strategy 109
practice development 81, 120, 150,
  154
  ~ precondition 29
practice gap 119
practice management system 123
practitioner 3, 6, 9, 23, 70,72, 73,
  74, 112, 125, 137
  ~ continuing development 35
  ~ ability to reflect 117
primary care groups 54, 83, 125,
  168
procedures 138
professional associations 170
professional development 161, 168
protocols 138
psychiatry 101

Q

qualitative 178, 181, 183
  ~ studies 185
qualitative research 183
quality 9, 66, 99, 111, 114, 117,
  151, 160, 164, 177,186, 189, 192